The Expectant Father:
The Ultimate Guide for Dads-to-Be

"For fathers soon expecting the ultimate gift—a new member of the family—*The Expectant Father* is his best friend."
—CNN Interactive

"One would be hard put to find a question about having a baby that's not dealt with here, all from the father's perspective."
—*Library Journal*

The New Father:
A Dad's Guide to the First Year

"This book would make a great gift for any new dad."
—Lawrence Kutner, Ph.D., columnist, *Parents* magazine

D1456264

"Read a book? Who has time? But you'd be wise to find some so you can take advantage of a fabulous resource... *The New Father.*"
—*Sesame Street Parents*

Fathering Your Toddler:
A Dad's Guide to the Second
and Third Years

"...Brott demystifies child development... and make[s] fathers...enjoy the vital role they play in their kids' lives even more. A great addition to any parenthood library."
—*Child* magazine

Father for Life:
A Journey of Joy, Challenge, and Change

"An essential guide for every dad."
—MSN.com

All titles available in e-book

ARMIN A. BROTT

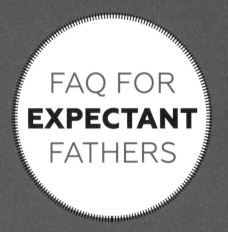

FAQ FOR
EXPECTANT
FATHERS

Abbeville Press Publishers
NEW YORK   LONDON

EDITOR: Will Lach
COPY EDITOR: Sharon Lucas
DESIGNER: Misha Beletsky
TYPESETTER: Ada Rodriguez
PRODUCTION MANAGER: Louise Kurtz

ISBN 978-0-7892-1269-6

Library of Congress Cataloguing-in-Publication Data available upon request

For bulk and premium sales and for text adoption procedures, write to Customer Service Manager, Abbeville Press,
116 West 23rd Street, New York, NY 10011,
or call 1-800-ARTBOOK.

Visit Abbeville Press online at
www.abbeville.com.

CONTENTS

INTRODUCTION

When I was an expectant father the first time, I had questions. Lots and lots of questions. And I became obsessed with finding answers. So I spent months doing research in libraries and I interviewed dozens of experts and hundreds of dads—some with more experience than I had, others with even less. What I discovered was that most guys—regardless of where they live, how much money they make, or whether they're a month into a first pregnancy or their child is 12 years old—have pretty much the same questions that I did.

My passion for finding answers ultimately led to my first book, *The Expectant Father.* Over the years, I've heard from thousands of expectant dads (and moms), and while they still crave information about those basic questions, some people want their answers in small, easily digestible chunks. That's why we created this series of FAQ books. Our goal is simple: to give you straightforward, solid answers to your most pressing questions, but in a fun, entertaining way that will help you retain the information so you can put it to use right away or recall it later on, whenever the need arises. Our test readers have loved this approach and we're confident that you will, too.

—Armin Brott
2016

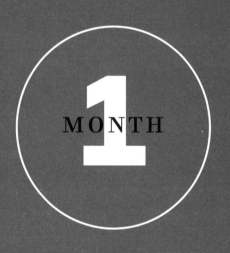

MONTH 1

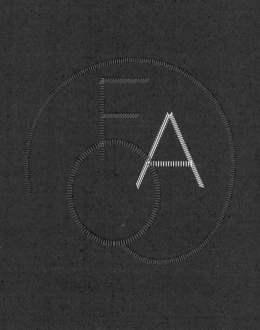

During the first trimester of the pregnancy, your partner needs about _____ more calories per day than before.

    a. 0
    b. 50
    c. 600
    d. 1200

a. In the first trimester, your partner needs about 0 more calories per day than before.

In the first trimester, your partner won't need to eat any more than usual—assuming she was a healthy weight before conceiving. In the second and third trimesters, though, she'll need about 300 extra calories per day.

TIP You can help her stay on track. If she was underweight before, she may need a little more, but if she's overweight, pregnancy is not the time to try to lose those extra pounds.

Women who have morning sickness are less likely to miscarry or deliver ____ .

a. mail
b. bad news
c. prematurely
d. a victory

c. Women who have morning sickness are less likely to miscarry or deliver prematurely.

Women who experience nausea and vomiting are less likely than those without symptoms to miscarry, deliver prematurely, or have low-birth-weight babies or babies with birth defects. In addition, some research has found that the more severe the mom's morning sickness, the higher the baby's IQ. Pregnant women over 35 who experience such symptoms benefit the most.

Once an egg is fertilized by a sperm, it becomes a _____ .

    a. baby chicken
    b. cell
    c. zygote
    d. nucleus

c. Once an egg is fertilized by a sperm, it becomes a zygote.

About two hours after sex, one very lucky sperm will have fertilized the egg, and, voilà, you've got yourself a zygote. By the end of the day, the zygote will divide into two cells and is now, technically, an embryo.

1 MONTH

Exercise during pregnancy improves _____ .

   a. the mother's running times

   b. the mother's strength and endurance

   c. the baby's muscle tone

   d. the baby's hearing

A

b. Exercise during pregnancy improves the mother's strength and endurance.

Exercising during pregnancy may steady your partner's weight gain, deepen her sleep, and lighten her mood. It also helps to improve strength and endurance, both of which will be useful during labor and delivery.

—

TIP If she needs a little extra motivation to exercise, work out with her.

A high- _____ diet supports the early surge in the baby's brain-cell growth.

    a. fat
    b. carb
    c. protein
    d. sugar

c. A high-**protein** diet supports the early surge in baby brain-cell growth.

Many medical professionals believe that a high-protein diet—especially during the first 19 weeks of pregnancy—supports the surge in the baby's brain-cell growth.

TIP Lean proteins are the best bet. Good sources include low-fat milk, tofu, and skinless chicken.

If your partner doesn't get enough iron, she may become _____ .

   a. Iron Man
   b. anemic
   c. depressed
   d. angry

b. If your partner doesn't get enough iron, she may become **anemic**.

Iron deficiency may cause anemia, which can leave your partner feeling exhausted, weak, pale, dizzy, or short of breath. She should try to get three servings of iron-rich foods per day. Spinach, dried fruits, beef, and legumes are all good sources.

TIP If her doctor prescribes iron supplements, be aware that they often cause constipation.

How many servings of fruits and vegetables should your partner have a day?

 a. 7
 b. 3
 c. 12
 d. 5

a. Your partner should have a total of at least 7 servings of fruits and vegetables a day.

TIP Key vitamins provided by fruits and vegetables include beta carotene, needed for your baby's cell and tissue development, vision, and immune system; vitamin C, crucial for your baby's bones and teeth, as well as the collagen in your baby's connective tissue; potassium, which helps control your partner's blood pressure; and folic acid, which helps prevent neural tube defects and promotes a healthy birth weight.

Your partner should try to drink at least 64 ounces of _____ per day.

    a. water
    b. milk
    c. soda
    d. vodka

A

a. Your partner should try to drink at least 64 ounces of **water** per day.

Staying hydrated is always a good idea. But it's especially important during pregnancy. Eight 8-ounce glasses of water per day is a good target—more if she's doing a lot of exercise or if she's pregnant during the summer. This will help her to replace the water she loses when she perspires, and to carry away waste products.

TIP Set a good example and drink plenty of water yourself.

Maternal _____ increases the risk of low-birth-weight babies and miscarriage.

a. laziness
b. mood swings
c. overeating
d. smoking

d. Maternal **smoking** increases the risk of low-birth-weight babies and miscarriage.

There's also strong evidence that exposing your partner and your baby to secondhand smoke is just as bad.

———

TIP If you or your partner hasn't quit smoking yet, this is the perfect time.

If your partner is vegetarian, she can still get the _____ she needs by eating healthy.

   a. nutrients
   b. meat
   c. eggs
   d. vegetables

A

a. If your partner is vegetarian, she can still get the **nutrients** she needs by eating healthy.

If your partner is a vegetarian, she and the baby can still get the nutrition they need by eating healthy foods—especially if she includes eggs and milk.

TIP If she's a strict vegan, you should check with her health-care provider or a nutritionist for special guidance.

Many men feel _____ upon finding out their partner is actually pregnant.

    a. angry and disgusted
    b. sad and lonely
    c. relieved and proud
    d. hungry and thirsty

c. Many men feel **relieved and proud** upon finding out their partner is actually pregnant.

Don't be surprised if you even feel proud of the fact that you're a stud!

However, if you're not the bio-logical father (say your baby was conceived with donor sperm), you're no less manly.

Your partner may be hungrier than usual, and you can help by _____ .

a. eating in front of her
b. buying lots of ice cream
c. preparing healthy meals
d. sending her to the store

c. Your partner may be hungrier than usual, and you can help by **preparing healthy meals**.

If your partner makes most of the meals, you can help make her life easier by taking over some of the shopping, meal planning, and preparation. Women are hungrier than usual during pregnancy, and eating healthy meals and snacks throughout the day is good for her and the baby.

TIP Learn to cook simple, nutritious meals and keep lots of healthy snacks around the house.

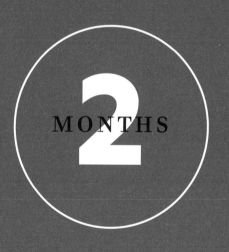

MONTHS

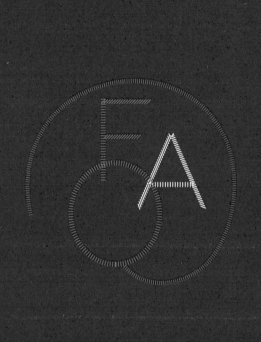

Early in pregnancy, mothers-to-be often worry about _____ , especially if you used assisted reproductive technology (ART).

    a. having twins
    b. miscarriage
    c. decorating the nursery
    d. choosing a nanny

b. Early in pregnancy, mothers-to-be often worry about **miscarriage**, especially if you used assisted reproductive technology (ART).

During the second month of the pregnancy, mothers-to-be may worry about the possibility of a miscarriage, especially if you used ART (which includes artificial insemination, egg donation, in-vitro fertilization, frozen embryo transfer, and donor sperm). At this stage of the pregnancy, they may also feel less attractive, have trouble staying focused, and experience temporary moodiness.

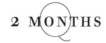
Studies show that women _____ with their pregnancies sooner than men.

    a. get annoyed
    b. connect
    c. become content
    d. rejoice

b. Studies show that women **connect** with their pregnancies sooner than men.

Although women can't feel the baby move yet, the physical changes they're experiencing make the pregnancy more "real" for them.

———

TIP The more you learn about the pregnancy and how the baby is developing, the sooner you'll connect. So keep reading this book!

2 MONTHS

For most men, pregnancy at two months is still _____ .

    a. a fairy tale
    b. an annoyance
    c. an abstract concept
    d. a surprise

c. For most men, pregnancy at two months is still an **abstract concept.**

Even though you may be excited about the pregnancy, you may forget for several days at a time that your partner is expecting. Just know, she *never* forgets.

You may find yourself trying not to get too excited about the pregnancy, in case of a _____ .

    a. set of triplets
    b. false pregnancy test
    c. miscarriage
    d. huge weight gain

c. You may find yourself trying not to get too excited about the pregnancy, in case of a **miscarriage**.

Many expectant dads make a conscious effort to stifle their excitement about their impending fatherhood. That way, if something goes wrong, they won't feel so devastated.

2 MONTHS

If your partner previously had a miscarriage, you may experience _____ of this pregnancy at first.

   a. denial
   b. excitement
   c. ignorance
   d. resentment

a. If your partner previously had a miscarriage you may experience **denial** of this pregnancy at first.

Dads who have been through a miscarriage on a previous pregnancy, or have done several unsuccessful ART cycles, are especially susceptible to self-protective (and completely understandable) denial.

_____ sexual desire is common during pregnancy, for both partners.

    a. Unusual
    b. Insatiable
    c. Increased
    d. Food-related

c. **Increased** sexual desire is common during pregnancy, for both partners.

During pregnancy, you may feel a newer, closer sexual connection to your partner. Some men feel this way because they're not worried about birth control anymore. Others may experience an increase in their feelings of masculinity, leading to a stronger sex drive.

———

TIP She really wants to hear that you find her beautiful.

2 MONTHS

Some men may experience a lack of _____ during pregnancy.

- **a.** food in the house
- **b.** sleep
- **c.** sexual attraction
- **d.** date nights

c. Some men may experience a lack of **sexual attraction** during pregnancy.

While some men's sex drive increases during pregnancy, others' may decrease. Some are turned off by their partner's changing body, or are afraid of hurting the baby. Others may even feel that sex is pointless now that she's finally pregnant.

TIP Unless you know that your partner is feeling the same way, keep these thoughts to yourself. Hearing that you don't find her attractive may make her think that you simply don't love her.

Many men deal with _____ by doing everything they can to get life back to normal.

a. pregnancy
b. infertility
c. grief
d. adoption

c. Many men deal with **grief** by doing everything they can to get life back to normal.

Expectant dads who've lost a baby often go back to work right away and put in longer-than-usual hours. It's a way of avoiding, coping, and—unfortunately—ignoring their feelings.

For many parents _____ is a second choice, made after many unsuccessful attempts to conceive.

    a. giving up
    b. starting a daycare
    c. adoption or surrogacy
    d. getting angry

c. For many parents, **adoption or surrogacy** is a second choice, made after many unsuccessful attempts to conceive.

Choosing to adopt a child or hire a surrogate is a decision many couples make only after years of unsuccessfully trying to conceive on their own, or after repeated disappointments and intrusive medical procedures.

2 MONTHS

Men who get involved early and stay involved are just as _____ the baby as their partner is.

- **a.** pregnant with
- **b.** connected with
- **c.** frustrated by
- **d.** ready for

b. Men who get involved early and stay involved are just as **connected with** the baby as their partner is.

The concept that women are connected to their pregnancy sooner than men has an exception: men who get involved early on and stay involved until the end have been shown to be as connected with the baby as their partners.

TIP The best way to stay involved is to read everything about pregnancy you can get your hands on (including, of course, this book).

Some men have trouble accepting the fact that they can't have their own _____ children.

    a. perfect
    b. biological
    c. wild
    d. adopted

A

b. Some men have trouble accepting the fact that they can't have their own **biological** children.

Talk to your partner about how you feel; she may be feeling a lot of similar things. The adoption agency you're working with most likely has a list of resources that can help you as well.

Expectant mothers typically go to the doctor once a _____ during the first trimester.

    a. month
    b. week
    c. day
    d. year

a. Expectant mothers typically go to the doctor once a **month** during the first trimester.

If your partner's pregnancy is progressing normally and is low risk, she'll typically continue to go to the doctor once a month through the end of the second trimester. The frequency will pick up in the third trimester.

Attending doctor appointments makes you more of a _____ , and less of a _____ .

    a. participant, spectator
    b. woman, man
    c. nice guy, jerk
    d. pushover, beast

a. Attending doctor appointments makes you more of a **participant**, and less of a spectator.

Going with your partner to as many of her medical appointments as possible is a great, concrete way to be an actively involved participant in the pregnancy.

———

TIP Going to the OB appointments is also a way to reassure your partner that you love her and are there for her.

A _____ is a noninvasive, painless procedure done any time after the fifth week of pregnancy.

a. urinalysis
b. paternity test
c. sonogram
d. heart transplant

c. A **sonogram** is a noninvasive, painless procedure done any time after the fifth week of pregnancy.

Your partner's health-care provider may order a sonogram (or ultrasound) any time after the fifth week of the pregnancy. By bouncing sound waves around the uterus and off the fetus, ultrasounds produce a picture of the baby and placenta.

TIP Don't miss this appointment—and ask the tech to print you a screen capture.

During your partner's pregnancy, you may want to be tested for _____ .

a. drugs
b. IQ
c. genetically transmitted birth defects
d. infertility

A

c. During your partner's pregnancy, you may want to be tested for **genetically transmitted birth defects.**

There may be times when you need to give a little blood to make sure all is well with your baby. A variety of genetically transmitted birth defects, for example, affect some ethnic groups more than others. Based on your family histories, your partner's doctor may suggest that one or both of you get additional blood tests done.

A(n) _____ is an accurate test that is usually performed between 15 and 18 weeks.

    a. baby sex test
    b. IQ test
    c. amniocentesis
    d. anemia screening

c. An **amniocentesis** is an accurate test that is usually performed between 15 and 18 weeks.

An amniocentesis can identify nearly every possible chromosomal disorder, including Down syndrome. It is also sometimes used in the third trimester to check the maturity of your baby's lungs.

TIP Even though this test is done on your partner, make sure to go with her. She may be feeling very nervous and will appreciate the support.

_____ is one of the most common pregnancy complications.

a. Preeclampsia
b. Heartburn
c. Miscarriage
d. Gestational diabetes

A

A. **Preeclampsia** is one of the most common pregnancy complications.

Preeclampsia is an increase in the mother's blood pressure that can deprive the fetus of blood and nutrients, and put the mother at risk for stroke or seizure. This dangerous condition affects about 10% of pregnant women. It usually happens in the last trimester but can appear at any time.

TIP You can't prevent preeclampsia, but you can reduce the risk by helping her exercise, cut back on salt, and get plenty of fiber.

Though men don't endure the physical pain of a miscarriage, they still experience _____ .

    a. the emotional pain
    b. the physical withdrawals
    c. nothing at all
    d. the abdominal cramping

a. Though men don't endure the physical pain of a miscarriage, they still experience **the emotional pain**.

Men's emotional pain after a partner's miscarriage can be just as severe as their partner's. Many men, like their partners, feel tremendous guilt and inadequacy when a pregnancy ends prematurely.

TIP If your partner does have a miscarriage, be there to support her emotionally. But make sure you get some support, too.

Sperm are on a(n) _____ day fertility cycle.

    a. every
    b. 90-
    c. 7-
    d. 30-

A

b. Sperm are on a **90-day** fertility cycle.

Women have fertility cycles—and so do men. Turns out that sperm are on a 90-day cycle, meaning that whatever happens to them today won't show up for three months.

TIP To improve sperm production and quality, don't spend too much time in hot tubs, don't sit with your legs crossed, and don't wear tight underwear.

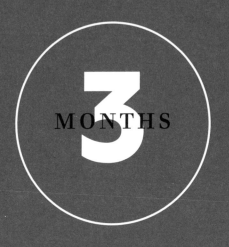

3
MONTHS

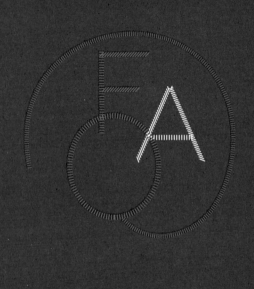

Fatigue and morning sickness usually start to _____ during the third month of pregnancy.

    a. peak
    b. disappear
    c. increase
    d. worsen

b. Fatigue and morning sickness usually start to **disappear** during the third month of pregnancy.

Many early pregnancy symptoms, including morning sickness, breast tenderness, and fatigue have all but disappeared by the end of the first trimester.

Though your partner doesn't look _____ , she may have trouble fitting into her clothes.

a. surprised
b. angry
c. irritated
d. pregnant

d. Though your partner doesn't look **pregnant**, she may have trouble fitting into her clothes.

She may have mixed feelings over her thickening waistline, frustrated one day and elated the next.

———

TIP The answer to "Do these jeans make my butt look big?" is always no.

3 MONTHS

The fetus looks like a _____ by the end of the third month.

   a. frog
   b. real person
   c. teenager
   d. blob

b. The fetus looks like a **real person** by the end of the third month.

At this point in the pregnancy, the fetus is only 2–3 inches long, weighs less than an ounce, has translucent skin, and a gigantic head. Other than that, she looks pretty much like a real person.

TIP "Gigantic" is a relative term. Your baby is about the size of a small apricot, and the head is about as big as a grape.

By the end of the third month of pregnancy, the baby will be able to curl his toes and even _____ .

    a. laugh
    b. snore
    c. tap dance
    d. frown

d. By the end of the third month of pregnancy, the baby will be able to curl his toes and even **frown**.

In addition, this month, your baby will develop all of his internal organs. Teeth, fingernails, toenails, and hair are coming along nicely, and so is the brain.

Hearing the baby's _____ for the first time can be a major reality booster.

    a. stomach growl
    b. laughter
    c. heartbeat
    d. brainwaves

c. Hearing the baby's **heartbeat** for the first time can be a major reality booster.

This month, the pregnancy begins to feel a little more tangible. At 120–180 beats per minute, the baby's heartbeat sounds more like a fast whoosh-whoosh-whoosh than an actual heart.

TIP Another appointment you don't want to miss. See if you can record the sound.

3 MONTHS

Many expectant fathers experience feelings of _____ during pregnancy.

    a. hunger
    b. ambivalence
    c. insanity
    d. exhaustion

b. Many expectant fathers experience feelings of **ambivalence** during pregnancy.

If you're feeling less than completely excited about the pregnancy, you're not alone. These feelings of ambivalence are often due to concerns over things like finances or whether you're adequately prepared to become a parent.

TIP Hang in there—you'll eventually get past this stage.

As your partner begins to bond more with the baby, you may feel left out or even _____ .

    a. relieved
    b. elated
    c. fickle
    d. jealous

d. As your partner begins to bond more with the baby, you may feel left out or even **jealous**.

During the third month, your partner may begin spending more time focusing on what is happening inside her body and establishing a bond with the baby. This may leave you feeling rejected or completely excluded.

***

TIP It's tempting, but don't try to get even by withdrawing from your partner. Instead, talk to her about how you're feeling.

Sometimes expectant dads are treated as onlookers or _____ by medical professionals.

    a. experts
    b. intruders
    c. cowboys
    d. buddies

A

b. Sometimes expectant dads are treated as onlookers or **intruders** by medical professionals.

Many men complain that medical professionals have a tendency to behave as if the expectant mother is the only one worth interacting with and the dad has no business being there.

TIP It's important to speak up and be assertive with your partner's health-care providers and let them know you want to be involved.

As many as _____ of American expectant fathers experience sympathetic pregnancy.

    a. 10%
    b. 30%
    c. 80%
    d. 75%

c. As many as 80% of American expectant fathers experience sympathetic pregnancy.

Various studies estimate that as many as 25–80% of American dads-to-be experience couvade syndrome, also known as sympathetic pregnancy.

TIP Don't be surprised if you experience food cravings, nausea, mood swings, and even weight gain.

3 MONTHS

Set aside _____ every day to talk with your partner about something—anything—other than the baby.

    a. 45 minutes
    b. 1 hour
    c. 15 minutes
    d. 5 minutes

c. Set aside 15 minutes every day to talk about something—anything—other than the baby.

I know this sounds awfully simple, but if you get into the habit now, while your life is still relatively calm, you'll be taking a huge step toward keeping your relationship fresh. It really does work, and making a commitment to doing it every day is absolutely critical. The more satisfied you feel in your relationship before you have children, the more time you'll spend with your child during the first year of her life.

3 MONTHS

Some men develop couvade symptoms as a way to shift the focus of pregnancy to _____ .

    a. the baby
    b. the mom
    c. the doctor
    d. themselves

d. Some men develop couvade symptoms as a way to shift the focus of pregnancy to **themselves**.

It's as if they're saying, "Hey, she's not the only one around here who can't fit into her pants." Similarly, physical symptoms can be a public way to assert paternity.

——

TIP Think about what's going on with you and your body. Have you noticed any changes that you can't really explain?

Telling other people about the pregnancy can make it seem more _____ .

   a. public
   b. interesting
   c. real
   d. exciting

c. Telling other people about the pregnancy can make it seem more **real**.

Many couples keep their pregnancy to themselves until they've gotten over their fears of miscarriage or other pregnancy disasters.

———

TIP Make sure you and your partner agree on when to spill the beans.

It's _____ for expectant siblings to insist that they, too, are pregnant like Mommy.

    a. uncommon
    b. rare
    c. not unusual
    d. ridiculous

c. It's **not unusual** for expectant siblings to insist that
they, too, are pregnant like
Mommy.

Insisting that they're not may
make them feel excluded and
resentful of the new baby. This
is especially true for little boys.

Expectant dads' levels of cortisol and prolactin _____ their partners'.

    a. are higher than
    b. parallel
    c. are less than
    d. have an impact on

A

b. Expectant dads' levels of cortisol and prolactin **parallel** their partners'.

Blood samples taken from expectant mothers and fathers at various points during the pregnancy found that expectant dads' levels of cortisol and pro-lactin (which you wouldn't think guys would even have) rise and fall along with their partners'.

When family members hear that you've decided to adopt or use ART, some of them may not _____ .

    a. understand
    b. care
    c. listen
    d. be too happy

d. When family members hear that you've decided to adopt or use ART, some of them may not **be too happy.**

Although you'd think that everyone would be overjoyed at your decision to adopt or use a donor, that's not always the case. Some people, especially relatives, might be disappointed or even resent that you're bringing an "outsider" into your family.

If you're not _____ , be ready for friends and family to ask when you'll take that step.

    a. a home owner
    b. living together
    c. married
    d. buying diapers

C. If you're not **married**, be ready for friends and family to ask when you'll take that step.

Even in the 21st century, when it's the norm for couples to live together before getting married, having a child out of wedlock still raises eyebrows in some circles. Your most liberal-minded friends and relatives may surprise you by suggesting that you "make an honest woman" out of your partner before the baby is born.

Expectant dads often feel that being strong for their partner means _____ how pregnancy affects them.

    a. telling everyone
    b. getting help for
    c. never acknowledging
    d. whispering

A

c. Expectant dads often feel that being strong for their partner means **never acknowledging** how pregnancy affects them.

We often try to protect our pregnant partners by minimizing the stress in their life. One way we do this is by not talking about our own concerns.

TIP She really, really wants to know what you're feeling. Not telling her may make her think you don't care and could hurt your relationship.

Before the baby is born, it's important to discuss what your involvement will be in _____ .

   a. family tasks
   b. space exploration
   c. meal preparation
   d. doctor appointments

a. Before the baby is born, it's important to discuss what your involvement will be in family tasks.

Long before the baby arrives, you and your partner need to have some serious discussions about division of labor around the house. How much does your partner expect you to do? How much do you expect her to do? It may sound harsh, but the reality is that you'll be as involved with your children only as much as your partner will let you be.

_____ are two major issues you and your partner should discuss before your baby arrives.

a. Eating and sleeping
b. Diaper duty and feedings
c. Names and nicknames
d. Religion and discipline

A

d. **Religion and discipline** are two major issues you and your partner should discuss before your baby arrives.

What, if any, religious education do you plan to give your child? How do you feel about spanking? It's better to talk about these things now, a little at a time, than to seethe about them for months and have some kind of explosion later.

Throughout the pregnancy, don't forget to talk about _____ .

   a. your partner's big belly
   b. how you're feeling
   c. politics
   d. your lack of interest

b. Throughout the pregnancy, don't forget to talk about how you're feeling.

Throughout the pregnancy, don't forget to talk about how you're feeling—good, bad, or indifferent. Talk about your excitement, fears, worries, and ambivalence.

TIP It's also important to ask your partner what she's feeling about the same things. As difficult as it may seem, learning to communicate with each other now will help you for years to come.

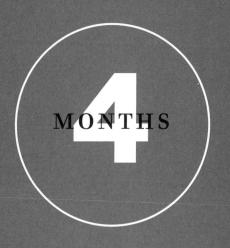

MONTHS

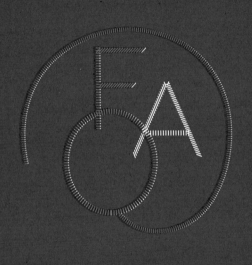

4 MONTHS

Sometime this month, your partner's _____ may begin to darken.

   a. eyes
   b. nipples
   c. fingernails
   d. mood

b. Sometime this month, your partner's **nipples** may begin to darken.

Increasing skin pigmentation during pregnancy can cause temporary darkening of your partner's nipples. Any freckles or moles she has may also be getting darker and more noticeable.

TIP Remind her that this is completely normal and makes her even more beautiful.

4 MONTHS

As her morning sickness subsides, she may regain her appetite for _____ .

    a. sex
    b. exercise
    c. pickles
    d. red wine

a. As her morning sickness subsides, she may regain her appetite for **sex**.

In the fourth month of pregnancy, many expectant mothers notice a significant decline in nausea from morning sickness. As a result, her appetite may begin to recover as well—for food and for sex.

4 MONTHS

Sixty to seventy-five percent of pregnant women have swollen, bleeding gums, which may be a sign of _____ .

    a. cavities
    b. overbrushing
    c. gingivitis
    d. yeast infection

c. Sixty to seventy-five percent of pregnant women
   have swollen, bleeding
   gums, which may be a sign
   of gingivitis.

During the fourth month of
pregnancy, your partner may
notice that her gums are more
sensitive than before. They may
be swollen, and even bleed at
times.

TIP Encourage her to keep
brushing and flossing—and to
ask her dentist whether a softer
brush might help.

Your partner may feel _____ when her regular clothes stop fitting her in the second trimester.

    a. excited
    b. fat
    c. anxious
    d. depressed

A

d. Your partner may feel **depressed** when her regular clothes stop fitting her in the second trimester.

While excited about her new "baby bump," your partner may feel depressed when her regular clothes stop fitting her, and may become nearly obsessed with her appearance.

TIP Remind her how much you love her—changing body and all—and how much you're looking forward to being a dad.

Sometime this month, the fetus
will be able to kick, swallow,
and _____ .

   a. suck his thumb
   b. drink milk
   c. shoot a 3-pointer
   d. laugh

a. Sometime this month, the fetus will be able to kick, swallow, and **suck his thumb**.

He can also respond to light and dark. A bright light shone on your partner's abdomen will cause him to turn away.

4 MONTHS

Talking about the baby and hearing her heartbeat will help the pregnancy seem more _____ .

    a. fun
    b. permanent
    c. real
    d. exciting

c. Talking about the baby and hearing her heartbeat will help the pregnancy seem more **real**.

Besides seeing the ultrasound, doing things like discussing the pregnancy with the mother and hearing the baby's heartbeat at medical appointments can make the pregnancy seem like it's really happening.

TIP Be patient—soon you'll be able to feel the baby move. That, too, can be a major reality booster for both parents.

It's not unusual to experience fear and anxiety over how you'll be able to _____ a baby.

    a. afford
    b. feed
    c. hold
    d. understand

a. It's not unusual to experience fear and anxiety over how you'll be able to **afford** a baby.

Once the fear of miscarriage has passed, many men find themselves faced with a new fear: How can we afford a new baby? This is especially true for fathers in their early and mid-twenties. Guys over 32 tend to be more settled in their careers, and usually have fewer concerns about money.

When commissioning a surro-gate, it's important to establish a _____ early on.

    a. credit line
    b. fee schedule
    c. name
    d. bond

A

d. When commissioning a surrogate, it's important to establish a **bond** early on.

The bond between a surrogate and the couple hiring her is sometimes referred to as a "forced friendship." Nevertheless, 98% of commissioning mothers and 90% of fathers rate their relationship with the surrogate mother as "harmonious."

Providing financially as a father is a form of _____ , even though many don't see it that way.

    a. retribution
    b. involvement
    c. torture
    d. pregnancy

A

b. Providing financially as a father is a form of **involvement**, even though many don't see it that way.

In some ways, work and fatherhood are inseparable. But very few people (except dads) see providing for the family as actual involvement. This may be because the act of providing is invisible, meaning that the work generally takes place away from the family.

TIP While bringing home the bacon is important, being an involved dad is going to mean a lot more than that.

Studies have shown that men go to the _____ much less often than usual when their partner is pregnant.

- **a.** casino
- **b.** bar
- **c.** doctor
- **d.** movies

c. Studies have shown that men go to the **doctor** much less often than usual when their partner is pregnant.

Many expectant fathers become preoccupied with the physical health and safety of their growing family, but they tend to ignore their own.

TIP The best way to help your family is to stay healthy. If you haven't had your annual physical or you need to see a doctor for any other reason, do it now, while life is still relatively calm.

If you're worried about your partner's health, encourage her to eat right, exercise, and _____ .

   a. ignore it
   b. smoke
   c. go hang gliding
   d. drink plenty of water

d. If you're worried about your partner, encourage her to eat right, exercise, and **drink plenty of water**.

If you feel overly concerned and protective of your partner and baby, try to relax a little. The most important thing you can do is encourage her to eat right, exercise, and drink plenty of water. Most of the rest will take care of itself.

TIP If you're still worried, discuss your concerns at her next doctor's appointment.

_____ when she says, "You have no idea what it's like to be pregnant."

    a. Smile and nod
    b. Argue
    c. Get angry
    d. Laugh

A

a. **Smile and nod** when she says, "You have no idea what it's like to be pregnant."

She's right, you know. While you may understand what pregnancy is like for you as a man, you'll never fully understand what's it's like for your partner.

TIP Someday, when you're sure it won't lead to a fight, you can tell her about what the pregnancy was like from your perspective.

In the last 20 years, college tuition and expenses have gone up _____ each year.

    a. 6–8%
    b. 20%
    c. very little
    d. 12%

a. In the last 20 years, college tuition and expenses have gone up **6–8%** each year.

College tuition and expenses, such as room and board, have gone up 6–8% per year—a lot faster than inflation. Most experts expect them to rise at about the same rate for years to come.

TIP It's important that you start planning for college now. Chances are, whatever you're planning to put aside for your child's education isn't going to be enough.

If she's up for it, a little bit of
_____ can help keep things
interesting.

    a. laundry
    b. cooking
    c. sexting
    d. talking

A

c. If she's up for it, doing a little bit of **sexting** can help keep things interesting.

There will be times when your partner feels less than attractive. If she's game, doing a little bit of sexting can add a spark to your relationship and remind her that you still find her desirable. It's not unusual for men to find themselves even more sexually drawn to their partner during pregnancy.

Your _____ during pregnancy has a big effect on the kind of mother your partner will be.

    a. diet
    b. IQ
    c. salary
    d. support

A

d. Your **support** during pregnancy has a big effect on the kind of mother your partner will be.

Supporting your partner during the pregnancy is absolutely critical. It has a concrete effect on her emotional and physical health, as well as on the kind of mother she'll be after the baby comes.

TIP The more you show her that you love her and are excited about being a dad, the happier she'll be.

A college graduate with a bachelor's degree earns about _____ than a high-school grad.

    a. 60% more
    b. 25% more
    c. 10% more
    d. 30% less

a. A college graduate with a bachelor's degree earns about **60**% more than a high-school grad.

People with a master's degree earn twice as much as those with only a high-school diploma.

TIP You're going to be plenty busy for the next few years, but think about whether getting another degree—or finishing your first one—makes sense for you and your family.

The more _____ your child has,
the _____ financial aid you'll be
eligible for.

    a. freckles, more
    b. assets, less
    c. assets, more
    d. friends, more

b. The more **assets** your child has, the **less** financial aid you'll be eligible for.

Schools assume that 35% of your child's assets will be available for educational purposes each year, but only 6% of yours.

A 529 plan is a type of _____ education savings account.

    a. grandparent-funded
    b. federally funded
    c. locally sponsored
    d. state-sponsored

d. A 529 plan is a type of **state-sponsored** education savings account.

The best option for most parents is a 529 plan. Contributions are made with after-tax dollars, but the earnings are completely exempt from federal taxes (and in most cases, state taxes as well).

There are _____ income restrictions on 529 savings plans.

    a. heavy
    b. no
    c. federal
    d. state

b. There are **no** income restrictions on 529 savings plans.

Unlike some other college savings plans (including Coverdell Educational Savings Accounts), 529 plans are especially attractive because they have no income restrictions. Plus the money can be used for tuition, books, room, and board at any accredited, post-high-school institution in the country.

———

TIP There are limits to how much you can sock away in a 529. Check with your plan's administrator to find out yours.

Wills, trusts, and health-care directives are all crucial to have in case of _____ .

    a. unexpected pregnancy
    b. an untimely death
    c. a loss of job
    d. divorce

b. Wills, trusts, and health-care directives are all crucial to have in case of an untimely death.

Planning for the unexpected is always important, but even more so when you have a family that depends on you. Having a will, trust, and health-care directive ensures that your wishes will be carried out in case of your (or your partner's) tragic, untimely death.

———

TIP Because every family's circumstances are different, get some advice from a probate attorney.

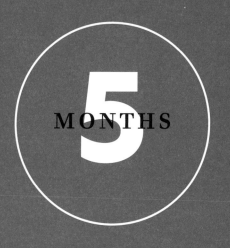

5

MONTHS

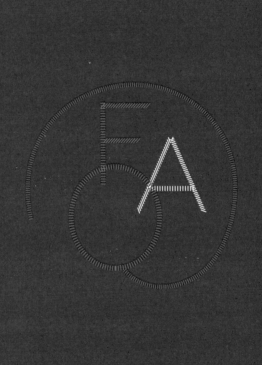

5 MONTHS

Your partner may begin to recognize more baby _____ during the fifth month.

    a. belly
    b. movement
    c. sounds
    d. names

b. Your partner may begin to recognize more baby **movement** during the fifth month.

This month, your partner will probably begin feeling more of the baby's movements. She may now actually recognize that that's what those fluttering feelings are.

TIP It may be a little too early for you to feel any of these movements. But just in case, ask your partner to place your hand on wherever the kicks seem to be coming from.

Painless, occasional tightening of the uterus is known as _____ .

   a. Braxton-Hicks contractions
   b. real labor
   c. cramping
   d. Toni Braxton contractions

a. Painless, occasional tightening of the uterus is known as **Braxton-Hicks contractions**.

Braxton-Hicks contractions, or "false labor," are named after the English obstetrician who "discovered" them back in the 19th century (although they existed long before he identified them). During real labor, the cervix begins to open; in false labor, it doesn't.

5 MONTHS

Expectant mothers may notice the appearance of a _____ from the belly button down the abdomen.

a. stretch mark
b. baby imprint
c. dark line
d. large scar

c. Expectant mothers may notice the appearance of a **dark line** from the belly button down the abdomen.

The *linea nigra* (Latin for "black line") typically makes its appearance about halfway through the pregnancy. It looks a little odd, but it's normal and harmless.

TIP If your partner is feeling self-conscious, don't make a big deal of this. It'll go away not long after the baby is born.

5 MONTHS

Many women notice a change
in their _____ due to fluid
retention.

    a. bathroom breaks
    b. biceps
    c. vision
    d. hip size

c. Many women notice a change in their **vision** due to fluid retention.

Pregnant women carry around about 50% more bodily fluids (mostly blood and water) than when they're not pregnant. Some of that excess fluid may change the shape of her eyeballs. If she wears contacts, they may irritate her or no longer fit. This is temporary and her eyeballs will return to their normal shape when the pregnancy is over.

5 MONTHS

_____ changes can cause for-getfulness, brittle nails, and splotchy skin.

a. Diet
b. Sleep
c. Hormone
d. Job

A

c. **Hormone** changes can cause forgetfulness, brittle nails, and splotchy skin.

Hormones are causing all sorts of trouble during this month. Your partner is forgetful, her fingernails may be brittle, and her skin may be splotchy.

TIP It's virtually impossible to tell her too many times that you love her and that she's beautiful.

Your partner will worry less about _____ once she can feel the baby move.

    a. miscarriage
    b. horseback riding
    c. labor
    d. gaining weight

A

a. Your partner will worry less about **miscarriage** once she can feel the baby move.

Most pregnant women feel reassured by the baby's movements and worry less about miscarriage. But those worries may come rushing back if those movements slow way down or stop altogether.

TIP During the day, when your partner is up and about, the baby is being rocked to sleep and will move less. Pay more attention to kicks when your partner is relaxing.

5 MONTHS

By month five, the baby's eye-brows and lashes are _____ .

    a. blonde
    b. thick
    c. still nonexistent
    d. fully grown

d. By month five, the baby's eyebrows and lashes are **fully grown**.

The baby's eyelids are still sealed, but the eyebrows and lashes are fully grown in. Your baby may even have some hair on the head.

Babies start having occasional bouts of _____ in the fifth month.

a. hiccups
b. karaoke
c. heartburn
d. diarrhea

A

a. Babies start having occasional bouts of **hiccups** in the fifth month.

Your baby may get the hiccups as often as several times a day. Your partner probably won't notice them for another month or two, but when she does, she'll tell you that they feel quite different than the baby's kicks.

Your baby is now able to _____ what's going on outside the womb.

    a. see
    b. feel
    c. know
    d. hear

A

d. Your baby is now able to **hear** what's going on outside the womb.

You can play soothing music and talk to your baby now, as she is able to hear what's going on outside the womb.

————

TIP If you aren't already talking to your baby, now's a great time to start. A few minutes a day, at the same time, will help your baby recognize your voice within hours after the birth.

Feeling the baby _____ for the first time is a big reality booster for expectant fathers.

a. kick
b. sing
c. dance
d. hiccup

A. Feeling the baby **kick** for the first time is a big reality booster for expectant fathers.

Even after seeing the baby on the sonogram and hearing the heartbeat, it can still be hard to believe you're going to be a father. But feeling the baby kick for the first time will pretty much remove any lingering doubts you may have had. After all, it's pretty hard to fake a kick.

You may find yourself wanting to spend more time with others who have _____ .

    a. big televisions
    b. teenagers
    c. small children
    d. no kids

c. You may find yourself wanting to spend more time with others who have small children.

As the pregnancy progresses, you may start spending more time with friends or relatives who have little kids, or you may find yourself watching strangers—especially men—interacting with their children.

TIP Pay close attention, and you'll probably notice a difference in the way younger fathers behave. And you'll definitely notice the differences between how moms and dads behave.

5 MONTHS

Your partner may feel _____ and need reassurance that you aren't going to leave.

    a. frustrated
    b. insecure
    c. angry
    d. indifferent

A

b. Your partner may feel **insecure** and need reassurance that you aren't going to leave.

As your partner's body continues to change, her hormones may have left her feeling insecure, emotionally needy, and craving confirmation that you love her and will always be there for her and the baby.

TIP Notice her subtle and not-so-subtle hints and give her the attention she needs. If you don't, she may think you don't care.

5 MONTHS

No matter how much _____ you do about pregnancy, you still may feel unprepared.

    a. talking
    b. praying
    c. watching
    d. reading

A

d. No matter how much **reading** you do about pregnancy, you still may feel unprepared.

At some point, it's going to hit you that in only a few short months, you'll be facing the biggest challenge of your life. Even with reading and taking classes about pregnancy, childbirth, and babies, you may still feel a little (or a lot) unprepared.

TIP Stick with us—by the time you finish this book, you'll be as ready as it's possible to be.

Fetuses can tell the difference between two _____ , and show preference for their native one.

    a. homes
    b. plants
    c. countries
    d. languages

d. Fetuses can tell the difference between two **languages**, and show preference for their native one.

Your baby isn't even born yet, but she's already learned to recognize what will be her native language. Newborns will stare longer at people speaking the language that their mother spoke during pregnancy than at those speaking a different language.

Prenatal _____ with your baby can help establish a bond even before birth.

 a. classes
 b. conversations
 c. exercises
 d. arguments

A

b. Prenatal **conversations** with your baby can help establish a bond even before birth.

You'll probably feel a little silly at first, but talking with (okay, talking *to*) your baby now is a great way to start getting to know each other. Within hours after the birth, when you say something to your baby, he'll recognize your voice and will turn to look at you.

TIP Set aside a few minutes every day (at the same time, if possible) and either talk to or read to your baby.

If you have to be gone for an extended period during the pregnancy, make a _____ of yourself reading or singing and ask your partner to play it for the baby.

a. mockery
b. recording
c. cake
d. portrait

b. If you have to be gone for an extended period during the pregnancy, make a **recording** of yourself reading or singing and ask your partner to play it for the baby.

If you travel a lot for work, or are deployed with the military, this is a great way for your baby to get to know your voice while you're gone.

TIP You can also read and talk to your baby through Skype or phone, just have your partner put the headset or speaker near her belly.

5 MONTHS

_____ can do funny things to
your libido, and you may find
yourself hornier than ever.

    a. Babies
    b. Weight gain
    c. Squirrels
    d. Pregnancy

d. **Pregnancy** can do funny things to your libido, and you may find yourself hornier than ever.

Some guys are more interested in sex than ever, while others are repelled by the idea. Same goes for the moms-to-be. The two of you may be feeling the same thing at the same time, or you may be on opposite ends of the sexual arousal scale. Either way, it's perfectly normal.

———

TIP If you and your partner aren't in sync, talk it over and try some nonsexual affection.

Increased _____ in the pelvic area may make your partner's orgasms more powerful and frequent.

    a. size
    b. flexibility
    c. blood flow
    d. penetration

A

c. Increased **blood flow** in the pelvic area may make your partner's orgasms more powerful and frequent.

During pregnancy, increased vaginal lubrication and blood flow to her pelvic area may make your partner's orgasms stronger and easier to achieve. This may prompt her to masturbate more than usual as well.

TIP There's no reason at all why you can't join in the fun. . . .

You or your partner may be afraid that _____ could hurt her or the baby.

    a. sexual activity
    b. bike riding
    c. hot baths
    d. roller coasters

a. You or your partner may be afraid that **sexual activity** could hurt her or the baby.

It can't. The baby is safely cushioned by its amniotic-fluid-filled sac, and unless your partner has cramps or bleeding, or the doctor has advised against it, sex during pregnancy is no more dangerous than at any other time.

5 MONTHS

Expectant fathers tend to be more inhibited about _____ than their partners.

   a. oral sex
   b. their body
   c. physical intimacy
   d. masturbation

c. Expectant fathers tend to be more inhibited about **physical intimacy** than their partners.

Expectant fathers have more psychological inhibitions about physical intimacy during pregnancy than their partners do. Most men find their pregnant partner's body erotic, but don't always tell her because they worry that she's not feeling attractive.

TIP If your partner's body makes you horny, tell her about it. What's the worst that could happen?

5 MONTHS

_____ affection during pregnancy is important for your relationship.

    a. Occasional
    b. Lack of
    c. Sexual
    d. Nonsexual

A

d. **Nonsexual** affection during pregnancy is important for your relationship.

Sex is an important part of your relationship with your partner. But during pregnancy, as your sex life changes, things like snuggling, hugging, and even just touching become just as important.

TIP Nonsexual affection can be misinterpreted as foreplay, so be sure to communicate your intent. If you offer a back rub, don't go any further than that unless she asks for more.

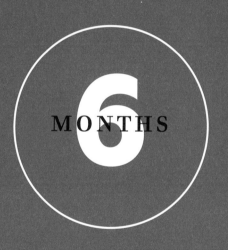

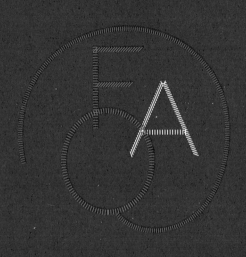

Expectant mothers often experience _____ leakage when laughing, coughing, or sneezing.

   a. milk
   b. saliva
   c. urine
   d. mucus

c. Expectant mothers often experience **urine** leakage when laughing, coughing, or sneezing.

Your partner's expanding, baby-filled uterus is putting pressure on her bladder. As a result, a little urine may leak out at the most inopportune—and potentially embarrassing—times.

TIP If this is happening to your partner, she'll be feeling plenty self-conscious, so skip any jokes about adult diapers.

6 MONTHS

The greatest period of _____ during pregnancy begins in the sixth month.

    a. weight gain
    b. frustration
    c. communication breakdown
    d. insomnia

A

a. The greatest period of **weight gain** during pregnancy begins in the sixth month.

Toward the end of the second trimester, most women begin to experience more rapid weight gain, as well as swelling of the hands and feet, and increased perspiration.

6 MONTHS

Your partner's heart and lungs are working _____ harder than before she was pregnant.

    a. 10%
    b. 50%
    c. 8%
    d. 25%

b. Your partner's heart and lungs are working 50% harder than before she was pregnant.

Thanks to all the excess blood, fluids, and other weight your partner is carrying around, her heart, lungs, and other organs are getting a real workout. Not surprisingly, everyday activities may leave her out of breath.

TIP Despite all this, she still needs to exercise—it builds strength and endurance and may make her labor shorter. If she's feeling sluggish, go out for walks together.

6 MONTHS

Expectant mothers often worry about how good a _____ they'll be.

a. wife
b. friend
c. person
d. parent

A

d. Expectant mothers often worry about how good a parent they'll be.

Your partner is probably spending a lot of time thinking about what kind of mother she'll be and whether the way she was mothered will affect her own parenting.

TIP Pay attention to what you're thinking, too—are you concerned about what kind of dad you'll be? Do you want to be just like him? The total opposite? Something in between?

6 MONTHS

Babies have their own unique
_____ and _____ before they're
born.

   a. footprints, fingerprints
   b. fingernails, toenails
   c. Social Security numbers,
      bank account numbers
   d. hair, eyes

A

a. Babies have their own unique **footprints** and **fingerprints** before they're born.

For the past few months, your baby has been using her hands and feet to explore the inside of the womb. The friction from all that touching has created ridges that are now your baby's unique finger- and footprints.

Your _____ has already had a profound influence on the kind of father you will be.

    a. best friend
    b. wife
    c. father
    d. education

c. Your **father** has already had a profound influence on the kind of father you will be.

You may find yourself flooded with forgotten images of childhood, especially ones involving your father.

———

TIP Whether your dad was a fantastic father or a not-so-great one, the father *you* become is 100% up to you.

6 MONTHS

You may begin thinking about your own _____ , and how it could affect those around you.

    a. lifestyle
    b. habits
    c. death
    d. job

c. You may begin thinking about your own **death**, and how it could affect those around you.

There's something about becoming a father that makes men begin contemplating their own mortality. Now that you have a family depending on you, you may worry about what would happen to your partner and child(ren) if something terrible were to happen to you.

It's common to experience a heightened sense of _____ to your relatives during pregnancy.

   a. attachment
   b. frustration
   c. awareness
   d. irritation

a. It is common to experience a heightened sense of **attachment** to your relatives during pregnancy.

All that thinking about your own father and your own mortality may make you feel a stronger connection to your relatives. A lot of expectant dads develop a keen interest in exploring their family tree.

6 MONTHS

As your partner becomes increasingly dependent on you, you may begin feeling _____ .

    a. confident
    b. angry
    c. offended
    d. trapped

A

d. As your partner becomes increasingly dependent on you, you may begin feeling trapped.

Besides being dependent on you, your partner needs a lot of reminding that you love her and are committed to being an involved dad. That puts a lot of pressure on you and can make you feel as though your own independence is being threatened.

TIP If you're feeling this way, be sure to talk to you partner about getting a little "me" time or spending some time with your buddies. Of course, you'll need to reciprocate.

6 MONTHS

Take lots of _____ during the pregnancy. You'll both regret it later if you don't.

    a. naps
    b. vacations
    c. sedatives
    d. pictures

d. Take lots of **pictures** during pregnancy. You'll both regret it later if you don't.

Many women are shy about having their picture taken while they're pregnant. But if you don't capture these moments, you'll regret it later on.

TIP Take pictures of your partner at least once a month, more often if she's up to it. Be sure to get front and side shots, and keep up with the dates.

6 MONTHS

A small percentage of mothers experience bizarre cravings, a condition known as _____ .

    a. gross
    b. pico de gallo
    c. pica
    d. porka

A

c. A small percentage of mothers experience bizarre cravings, a condition known as **pica**.

Food cravings during pregnancy are normal, although the combinations may sometimes seem strange. However, some women crave bizarre things like paint, ashes, wax, even cigarette butts. Needless to say, this is *not* normal behavior.

TIP If you notice your partner eating anything that isn't actually food, discuss it with her doctor right away.

Contrary to common stereo-types, trying to balance _____ isn't just a women's issue.

    a. a checkbook
    b. the scales
    c. work and family
    d. pros and cons

c. Contrary to common stereotypes, trying to balance **work and family** isn't just a women's issue.

In fact men are slightly more likely than women to experience work-family pressure. Over 80% of working fathers report at least some work-versus-family conflict.

———

TIP Have some conversations with your partner now—before the baby comes—about what the ideal work-family situation would be for your family.

6 MONTHS

During pregnancy, women's brains get 3–5% _____ .

    a. fatter
    b. smarter
    c. larger
    d. smaller

A

d. During pregnancy, women's brains get 3–5% smaller.

This is due to compression from extra blood, not actual loss of cells, and it goes back to normal within a few months after the birth.

———

TIP It's a good idea to keep this bit of knowledge to yourself. (Although since her brain is smaller, she might not remember—but if she does, you're in big trouble.)

_____ fathers consider family to be the most important aspect of their lives.

    a. Irresponsible
    b. Fully 75% of
    c. Gorilla
    d. Ignorant

b. Fully 75% of fathers consider family to be the most important aspect of their lives.

In fathers age 21–39, 70% say they'd give up some pay to be home more with their families, and 68% would consider being a stay-at-home parent if money were no object.

TIP Take a look at your family budget. Could you quit your job and become an at-home parent?

6 MONTHS

Only about 10% of new dads take more than _____ off after the birth of their child.

    a. 1 day
    b. 1 week
    c. 1 month
    d. 2 weeks

A

d. Only about 10% of new dads take more than **2 weeks** off after the birth of their child.

Unfortunately, men who take time off for family reasons are often viewed as not being serious about their job. Many men choose not to take time off simply because they feel it will hurt their career.

———

TIP Check with your company's HR department to see what benefits they offer new parents.

At least _____ of fathers work more than 40 hours per week, compared to 36% of mothers.

   a. 50%
   b. 25%
   c. 65%
   d. 80%

c. At least **65**% of fathers work more than 40 hours per week, compared to 36% of mothers.

Sadly, men who leave work to care for a newborn are rated much more negatively than those who don't. Compared to mothers, fathers are only one-tenth as likely to use parenting leave—even if it's paid.

———

TIP Look into your leave options now. Talk to your HR department—you may be surprised at what's actually available.

Businesses lose more than _____ a year as a direct result of over-worked, overstressed dads.

    a. $150 billion
    b. $1 million
    c. $500 million
    d. $1 billion

a. Businesses lose more than **$150 billion** a year as a direct result of overworked, overstressed dads.

Absenteeism, "presenteeism," employee turnover, excessive use of sick days, and unnecessary workers' comp claims from overworked, overstressed dads cost businesses $150 billion every year.

TIP When talking with your boss about taking time off after the baby comes, mention this statistic. Supporting you could actually help the bottom line.

There are at least _____ stay-at-home dads, and that number is growing daily.

a. 2 million
b. 5,000
c. 2 billion
d. 500,000

a. There are at least **2 million** stay-at-home dads, and that number is growing daily.

If your partner has a more stable career, makes more money than you, or simply has no interest in staying home, you may want to consider taking over the caregiver role.

Being a stay-at-home dad can be
_____ , and about two-thirds feel
isolated.

    a. lonely
    b. profitable
    c. educational
    d. exciting

A

a. Being a stay-at-home dad can be **lonely**, and about two-thirds feel isolated.

Being a stay-at-home parent of either sex isn't easy, but men who do it are twice as likely as women to feel isolated. Unfortunately, there just isn't a lot of social support available for men who choose this kind of non-traditional path.

TIP If you're considering being an at-home dad, check the National At-Home Dad Network (www.athomedad.org), which is a fantastic resource. There are more out there than you'd think.

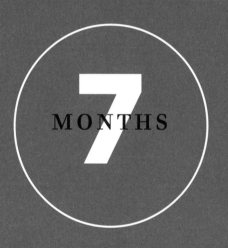

MONTHS

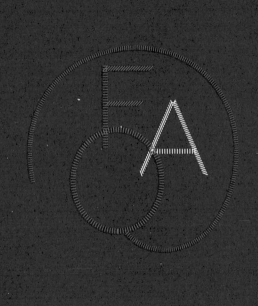

7 MONTHS

You're in the home stretch now! Your partner's hip joints are expanding, and she may _____ in a new, awkward way.

    a. pee
    b. have sex
    c. sit
    d. walk

d. You're in the home stretch now! Your partner's hip joints expand, and she may **walk** in a new, awkward way.

During the last trimester, your partner's hip joints will begin to expand to make room for the baby to move down during labor. Besides walking like a duck, she may be more susceptible to muscle pulls and general klutziness.

———

TIP Keep the penguin, duck, and waddling jokes to a minimum.

Toward the end of the pregnancy, mothers may notice a thick, white, yellowish or greenish white _____ called leukorrhea.

    a. vegetable
    b. lump
    c. vaginal discharge
    d. pimple

c. Toward the end of the pregnancy, mothers may notice a thick, white, yellowish or greenish white **vaginal discharge** called leukorrhea.

This is a result of her increased estrogen levels, and it's perfectly normal.

At this point, your partner may begin to feel fearful about _____ .

    a. takeout
    b. clothes
    c. labor and delivery
    d. the economy

A

c. At this point, your partner
   may begin to feel fearful
   about **labor and delivery**.

While your partner has been
pretty used to the idea of having
a baby for several months now,
the fact the she's actually going
to go through labor can be scary.

TIP One of the best things you
can do for her right now is make
sure she knows that you're in
this together and that you'll be
there to support her every step
of the way.

This month, your baby's eyes can fully open, and her _____ react to light and dark.

    a. brains
    b. pupils
    c. eyelids
    d. muscles

b. This month, your baby's eyes can fully open, and her **pupils** react to light and dark.

Your baby's lungs are also continuing to develop, and if she were born today, she'd have an excellent chance of survival.

Many men don't experience their children as completely real until they see them _____ .

a. cry
b. playing
c. face-to-face
d. sleep

c. Many men don't really experience their children as completely real until they see them **face-to-face**.

Despite hearing the baby's heartbeat, seeing the sonogram, and feeling the kicks, many men have trouble wrapping their head around the idea that an actual baby is in there.

TIP Start clearing your calendar to make sure you'll be at the birth.

When envisioning their baby, _____ of expectant fathers picture a 3- to 5-year-old child.

    a. 50%
    b. more than 90%
    c. 20%
    d. 75%

b. When envisioning their baby, **more than 90% of** expectant fathers picture a 3- to 5-year-old child.

When asked to describe themselves with their baby, expectant fathers talk about holding hands, riding bikes, playing catch, or doing something else interactive. Mothers almost always see themslves with a newborn.

———

TIP Read up on child development—it will help you keep your expectations reasonable. No matter how hard you wish for it, your baby won't be able to kick a ball back to you for at least a year.

Some say you can predict the baby's _____ by the mom's cravings, complexion, or hair growth.

a. shoe size
b. sex
c. birth dates
d. eye color

b. Some say you can predict the baby's **sex** by the mom's cravings, complexion, or hair growth.

Your partner's complexion, cravings, hair growth, weight gain, whether she's carrying the baby high or low or wide, are all examples of supposed ways to know if you are having a boy or girl. None are more reliable than a coin toss.

TIP If you figure out a sex-predicting technique that doesn't involve a sonogram and is right more than half the time, patent it now. You'll make a mint.

Some expectant fathers are afraid of getting a child of the _____ .

    a. dark side
    b. wrong sex
    c. ex-boyfriend
    d. wrong size

A

b. Some expectant fathers are afraid of getting a child of the **wrong sex**.

Many expectant fathers worry that they won't have the parenting experience they imagined or that they won't know what to do with a girl.

TIP Try to keep this kind of thinking to a minimum. Do you really want your baby to start off life as a disappointment to dad?

Fathers of _____ visit the nursery more often and stay longer than fathers of _____ .

    a. twins, triplets
    b. boys, girls
    c. girls, boys
    d. dogs, cats

b. Fathers of **boys** visit the nursery more often and stay longer than fathers of girls.

Boys tend to bring fathers into the family more. Fathers of newborn boys actually visit the nursery more often and stay there longer than fathers of girls.

Some men worry that playing physically with their daughter would somehow be _____ .

   a. fun
   b. boring
   c. hurtful
   d. inappropriate

d. Some men worry that playing physically with their daughter would somehow be **inappropriate**.

Some men feel uncomfortable with the idea of wrestling with their daughters.

———

TIP Wrestling with your daughter is not only safe and appropriate, it's also quite beneficial. Girls who do a lot of physical play with dad are more confident, less likely to become teen parents and more likely to be successful in their careers.

Many men dread labor because they don't want to see their partner _____ .

a. naked
b. have a baby
c. in pain
d. bleeding

A

c. Many men dread labor because they don't want to see their partner **in pain**.

As provider-protectors we instinctively want to do everything we can to stop our loved ones' pain. But childbirth causes pain that we can't do anything about, and that can leave us feeling helpless.

TIP Learn as much as you can about labor and delivery. The more you know, the better you'll be able to help your partner cope.

When choosing your baby's
_____ , watch out for strange
combinations of _____ .

    a. wardrobe, colors
    b. pets, fish
    c. crib, sheets
    d. name, initials

A

d. When choosing your baby's **name**, watch out for strange combinations of initials.

Before you make your final baby-name decision, think about what your child's initials could spell, especially in the age of texting and tweeting.

TIP Do you really want to saddle your kid with initials like OMG, LOL, TMI, or WTF?

Over _____ of fathers-to-be are present at the birth of their children.

    a. 90%
    b. 10%
    c. 50%
    d. 65%

A. Over **90**% of fathers-to-be are present at the birth of their children.

The percentage of fathers who are present for the birth of their children has been rising steadily for the past few decades. That's true regardless of race or socio-economic status.

Lamaze, Bradley, Leboyer, Dick-Read, and McMoyler are all different _____ .

    a. automobile races
    b. sexual positions
    c. childbirth methods
    d. children's authors

c. Lamaze, Bradley, Leboyer, Dick-Read, and McMoyler are all different **childbirth methods**.

Taking classes can reduce your fears about childbirth; the more you know, the more in control you'll feel. Lamaze and Bradley are the two most common methods, although there are others.

TIP When choosing a childbirth method, make sure to find out their stance on the father. Some methods all but leave dads out. This is a big day for you, too.

Some parents opt to donate or store their baby's _____ , which is a rich source of stem cells.

    a. amniotic sac
    b. teeth
    c. dirty diapers
    d. cord blood

d. Some parents opt to donate or store their baby's **cord blood**, which is a rich source of stem cells.

The blood inside the umbilical cord has been used to treat dozens of diseases.

––––

TIP If your family has a history of leukemia or other cancer, consider a private cord blood bank. But they're not cheap. If you don't go that route, donate the cord blood to a public bank so someone else can benefit. It's usually free and your OB or hospital staff will give you the details.

A _____ is trained to be there for both partners during labor, physically and emotionally.

    a. physical trainer
    b. lawyer
    c. midwife
    d. doula

d. A **doula** is trained to be there for both partners during labor, physically and emotionally.

You have the option to hire a doula for extra support during labor. A doula won't take your place as the father, but instead will be there to provide encouragement and support for both parents.

TIP If you do opt for a doula, remember that she's there for you, too.

Not every father feels the need to be (or even should be) present in the _____ .

    a. hospital cafeteria
    b. classroom
    c. delivery room
    d. child's life

A

c. Not every father feels the need to be (or even should be) present in the **delivery room**.

As many as half of all fathers feel ambivalent about participating in childbirth. Discuss your fears with your partner, but be aware that she may take your reluctance as a sign that you don't care about her or the baby.

TIP Unless there's a real medical reason for you not to be there, put your partner first. No one can support her as well as you can.

Even though military dads get _____ , sometimes it's trumped by the needs of the military.

    a. bonus baby allowance
    b. paternity leave
    c. labor and delivery pay
    d. a year off

b. Even though military dads get **paternity leave**, sometimes it's trumped by the needs of the military.

While the military offers paternity leave, exactly how much you'll be able to take is impossible to know. It doesn't count against your regular leave, but depending on your mission, there's no guarantee you'll actually be able to be there for the big day.

———

TIP If you know you won't be able to be there in person, check with command about other options (and read the next question for some specific ideas).

7 MONTHS

_____ is an alternative option for dads who can't be present in the delivery room.

a. Picking another day
b. Hanging with friends
c. Videoconferencing
d. Hiring a photographer

c. **Videoconferencing** is an alternative option for dads who can't be present in the delivery room.

If the hospital will allow it, and your partner is comfortable with it, you can set up a real-time phone or videoconference for the delivery. More than one deployed dad has seen his baby born via Skype. Really.

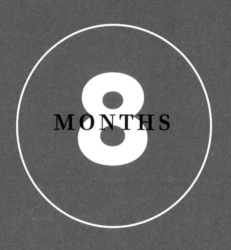

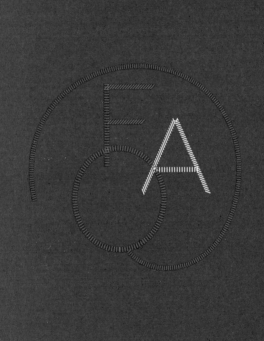

8 MONTHS

Braxton-_____ contractions become more frequent in the eighth month.

- **a.** Huckaby
- **b.** Bicks
- **c.** Bucks
- **d.** Hicks

d. Braxton-**Hicks** contractions become more frequent in the eighth month.

False labor contractions and a high level of general discomfort are among the many physical symptoms your partner will be experiencing from now through the end of the pregnancy.

———

TIP You can tell the difference between Braxton-Hicks contractions and real contractions. If they're getting stronger, longer, and closer together, they're the real deal.

8 MONTHS

As they get close to the end of the pregnancy, many mothers worry about their _____ in public.

    a. parking spaces
    b. water breaking
    c. baby being born
    d. sweaters fitting

b. As they get close to the end of the pregnancy, many mothers worry about their **water breaking** in public.

Expectant mothers have no control over when the amniotic sac will rupture, also known as "water breaking." Fortunately, it rarely happens in public.

8 MONTHS

Strangers may come up and
_____ your partner's belly
without bothering to ask for
permission.

    a. touch
    b. prod
    c. lick
    d. paint

A

a. Strangers may come up and **touch** your partner's belly without bothering to ask for her permission.

Something about a pregnant woman's belly seems to shout, "Touch me!" And lots of strangers will do just that.

TIP You may feel like popping someone in the nose for being so rude, but take your cues from your partner. If she's okay with it, let it go. If she's bothered by it, it's okay for her (or you) to politely tell people to keep their hands to themselves.

8 MONTHS

Sleeplessness, increased fatigue, and frequent _____ are common in this month.

    a. blindness
    b. urination
    c. nausea
    d. takeout meals

b. Sleeplessness, increased fatigue, and frequent **urination** are common in this month.

Your partner may also feel short of breath more often, as the baby is growing and your growing baby is pressing against her internal organs.

8 MONTHS

Most babies assume the _____ position sometime this month, and stay that way until birth.

   a. kickoff
   b. pike
   c. head-down
   d. feet-first

c. Most babies assume the **head-down** position sometime this month, and stay that way until birth.

If they're breech (feet or butt down) or transverse (shoulder or back down), there's still time for them to turn, but it's something your partner's medical provider will keep an eye on.

In the third trimester, your baby's heart is pumping around _____ of blood a day.

    a. 20 quarts
    b. 300 gallons
    c. 2,000 gallons
    d. 500 quarts

b. In the third trimester, your baby's heart is pumping around **300 gallons** of blood a day.

That may sound like a lot, but it's only a fraction of the 2,000 gallons that the average adult heart pumps daily.

8 MONTHS

Some couples use the last few months of pregnancy to _____ , since this may be their last chance for a long, long time.

    a. do housework
    b. get new jobs
    c. paint the house
    d. go on dates

A

d. Some couples use the last few months of pregnancy to **go on dates**, since this may be their last chance for a long, long time.

After a new baby is born, it'll be at least a few months (possibly years) before your social life gets back to normal. So have fun by going out together or with friends now, while you still can.

———

TIP Look into a "babymoon," a short getaway for expectant couples, usually featuring massage and other spa treatments (mostly for her).

8 MONTHS

Almost all expectant fathers experience some sort of _____ instinct.

    a. feeding
    b. betting
    c. nesting
    d. pregnancy

c. Almost all expectant fathers experience some sort of **nesting** instinct.

Although we think of nesting as a mom-to-be thing, most expectant dads go through something very similar.

———

TIP Activities like putting together cribs, painting the nursery, or installing the car seat are great ways you can prepare for your new child.

While sex in the second trimester is great, your sex life during the third trimester is bound to _____ .

    a. be 100 times better
    b. suffer
    c. be nonexistent
    d. stay the same

b. While sex in the second trimester is great, your sex life during the third trimester is bound to **suffer**.

No matter how hot and heavy your love life got in the second trimester, it's unlikely that things will continue at that pace. That's usually due to a combination of your partner's physical discomfort and a fear (yours or hers) of either hurting the baby or triggering premature labor.

———

TIP If you haven't already done so, now's a really good time to discuss nonsexual ways of connecting with your partner.

A _____ outlines your and your partner's goals and wishes for labor and delivery.

a. text message
b. power of attorney
c. birth plan
d. trust fund

c. **A birth plan** outlines your and your partner's goals and wishes for labor and delivery.

Spend some time talking about how you'd like labor and birth to go. Does she want an unmedicated, natural birth? Will she want the lights on or off? How does she feel about fetal monitoring? Will you want to be in the room if there's an emergency C-section?

TIP Remember, labor rarely goes as planned, so don't be so rigid that you alienate the medical team.

If you want to _____ when your baby is born, be sure to let the medical team know ahead of time.

   a. light up a cigar
   b. make a toast
   c. leave the room
   d. cut the umbilical cord

A

d. If you want to **cut the umbilical cord** when your baby is born, be sure to let the medical team know ahead of time.

Most dads want to cut the baby's umbilical cord right after the birth. But things can move awfully quickly, and if you haven't made your wishes clear in advance, the doctor may make the cut.

If the baby's head is too big, the doctor may do an episiotomy, a small surgical cut in the _____ .

    a. perineum
    b. stomach
    c. uterus
    d. ovaries

a. If the baby's head is too big, the doctor may do an episiotomy, a small surgical cut in the **perineum**.

If your partner's vagina won't stretch enough to allow the baby's head through, the doctor may suggest an episiotomy. This involves making a small cut in the perineum, the space between the vagina and anus, to make more room for the head to pass through.

TIP Try not to wince when you hear the word *episiotomy*.

Unless the doctor has told your partner otherwise, _____ in the third trimester is perfectly fine.

    a. sex
    b. motorcycle stunts
    c. frequent drinking
    d. smoking pot

a. Unless the doctor has told your partner otherwise, **sex** in the third trimester is perfectly fine.

Often times, one or both partners are afraid of hurting (or even poking) the baby during sex. Unless your partner's doctor has told you otherwise, sex in the third trimester poses no physical risk to the baby or your partner. That said, your partner may be getting to the point where having sex is too uncomfortable.

_____ at the hospital in advance saves time, and may even be required.

a. Sleeping
b. Registering
c. Paying
d. Touring

b. **Registering** at the hospital in advance saves time, and may even be required.

Most hospitals will allow, or may even require, you to register up to 60 days before the anticipated birth of your child. This isn't a reservation for a specific date; it just means that all of your partner's information is already in the system, which will save time when the big day finally comes.

8 MONTHS

It's important to start thinking now about the _____ you'll see once the baby is born.

    a. diapers
    b. bubble bath
    c. baby food
    d. pediatrician

d. It is important to start thinking now about the **pediatrician** you will see once the baby is born.

You don't actually have a baby yet, but you will soon, so it's important to start putting some real thought into selecting a pediatrician.

TIP Start by finding out which pediatricians are affiliated with the hospital where your baby will be born. Interview at least two different docs and bring a list of important questions.

8 MONTHS

Clothes, camera, chargers, and change are all things you should pack in your own _____ .

   a. vacation luggage
   b. trunk
   c. hospital bag
   d. Christmas presents

c. Clothes, camera, chargers, and change are all things you should pack in your own **hospital bag**.

Mothers aren't the only ones who need hospital bags. Once labor starts, you may not have a chance to get home for a few days, so in addition to your toothbrush and a change of clothes, be sure to pack your phone, camera, chargers, and change (for vending machines).

Don't forget to bring your baby's _____ with you, because the hospital won't let you take your baby home without one.

    a. diaper bag
    b. bottle
    c. Sunday best
    d. car seat

d. Don't forget to bring your baby's **car seat** with you, because the hospital won't let you take your baby home without one.

Actually, don't just bring the car seat—make sure it's installed according to the manufacturer's directions and that you know how to take it out and put it back in.

———

TIP Many local police and fire departments have car-seat clinics where they'll teach you to properly install one.

About 10% of babies are born
_____ , meaning sometime
before the 37th week.

    a. overweight
    b. late
    c. prematurely
    d. underweight

c. About 10% of babies are born **prematurely**, meaning sometime before the 37th week.

On average, a pregnancy lasts 40 weeks. A baby born anytime before the 37th week is considered premature. Depending on how early the baby comes, preemies may need to stay in the hospital a little longer and may experience health problems, some of which may last a lifetime. The earlier the birth, the more severe those problems are likely to be.

Premature labor symptoms are _____ those of real labor—they just happen before they should.

    a. the same as
    b. worse than
    c. less noticeable than
    d. completely different than

a. Premature labor symptoms are **the same as** those of real labor—they just happen before they should.

If your partner is experiencing premature labor symptoms, she should go to the hospital right away.

———

TIP Remember, if the contractions are getting longer, stronger, and closer together, they're real.

A(n) _____ means that the cervix is too weak and may open, resulting in premature labor.

    a. episiotomy
    b. incompetent cervix
    c. cervical spine
    d. ectopic pregnancy

A

b. An **incompetent cervix** means that the cervix is too weak and may open, resulting in premature labor.

The cervix connects the uterus to the vagina and keeps the baby inside the uterus until she's ready to be born. Cervical insufficiency, or incompetent cervix, occurs in 1–2% of pregnancies. It's usually diagnosed in the second trimester, but it may not be caught until the third trimester, especially in first pregnancies. The most common treatment is to sew the opening of the cervix shut. The sutures will be removed 2–4 weeks before the baby's due date.

Women who are _____ more than 5 hours a day are 3 times more likely to deliver prematurely.

    a. texting
    b. on their feet
    c. upside down
    d. on their butts

b. Women are on their feet more than 5 hours a day are 3 times more likely to deliver prematurely.

Women who work during pregnancy generally have fewer complications. However, spending long periods standing may increase the risk of premature delivery. It may also slow the baby's growth.

———

TIP Encourage her to take it easy. You may have to take on a bit more of the cooking and other household tasks so she can put her feet up for a few minutes. Plus, you're earning extra points. . . .

8 MONTHS

A baby's lungs aren't fully developed until at least the _____ week of the pregnancy.

   a. 20th
   b. 35th
   c. 28th
   d. 40th

c. A baby's lungs aren't fully developed until at least the **28th** week of the pregnancy.

Babies born before 28 weeks have a far higher risk of developing serious respiratory problems. Babies born at 28–32 weeks are far better off, but are still at risk for vision and gastrointestinal problems.

A crib, mattress, monitor, swing, and playpen are items you may want for the baby's _____ .

    a. birthday
    b. hospital room
    c. siblings
    d. nursery

A

d. A crib, mattress, monitor, swing, and playpen are items you may want for the baby's nursery.

Planning a nursery can be challenging. There are so many items to choose from, it's easy to feel overwhelmed. Focus on the items listed above (plus diapers, wipes, and a changing table), and you'll be okay.

8 MONTHS

_____ is a healthier, easier, and cheaper alternative to formula.

    a. Soda
    b. Cow's milk
    c. Breastfeeding
    d. Soy milk

c. **Breastfeeding** is a healthier, easier, and cheaper alternative to formula.

Breastfeeding is, without a doubt, the best thing for your baby. However, some mothers may have difficulty, or may choose not to breastfeed. Be sure to discuss these and other contingencies with your baby's health-care provider before the baby is born.

If your partner is worried about breastfeeding or has any questions or concerns, set up a meeting with a lactation consultant.

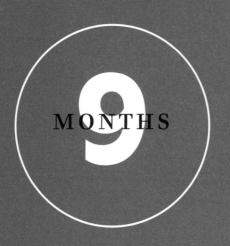

9 MONTHS

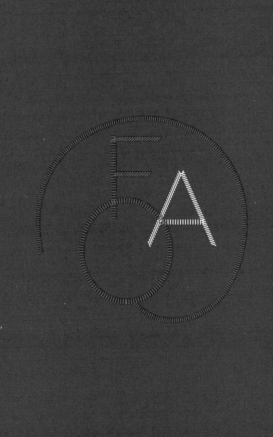

Your baby will go through about _____ diapers in the first year.

   a. 3,000
   b. 1,000,000
   c. 15,000
   d. 500

a. Your baby will go through about **3,000** diapers in the first year.

Now all you have to do is decide between cloth, disposable, compostable, biodegradable, and flushable. If you take everything into consideration (raw materials, resources used, pollution generated, and so on), the carbon footprints are, surprisingly, pretty much the same.

———

TIP If you keep your eye out for coupons and buy in bulk, there's not much price difference between cloth and disposables.

9 MONTHS

In the ninth month, the baby is so cramped that instead of kicking, all she can do is _____ .

    a. cry
    b. punch
    c. poke
    d. squirm

A

---

d. In the ninth month, the baby is so cramped that instead of kicking, all she can do is **squirm**.

Fortunately, babies aren't claustrophobic. In her last weeks of captivity, your baby will practice hand clenching, swallowing, head turning, and even breathing.

Your partner may feel a renewed sense of energy when the baby _____ .

    a. drops
    b. is born
    c. gets bigger
    d. sleeps more

A

a. Your partner may feel a renewed sense of energy when the baby **drops**.

About a month before birth, the baby's head (if he's in a head-down position) drops into the mom's pelvis, taking some of the pressure off her lungs and stomach.

9 MONTHS

Some mothers with older kids are afraid they won't have enough _____ to go around once the new baby is born.

    a. money
    b. breasts
    c. milk
    d. love

A

d. Some mothers with older kids are afraid they won't have enough love to go around once the new baby is born.

You may not fall in love with your baby right away, but eventually you will. And you'll find that it's a very different kind of love than you've ever felt—one many new parents worry they won't ever be able to replicate with a new baby.

TIP Love is not a zero-sum game. It's like lighting one candle with another—now you have two flames burning equally brightly.

_____ put on about a quarter to a half pound a week during the last month of pregnancy.

a. Mothers
b. Fathers
c. Babies
d. Piglets

c. **Babies** put on about a quarter to a half pound a week during the last month of pregnancy.

Babies slap on a lot of weight during the last month of pregnancy, but they usually stop growing about a week before birth. Average babies weigh 6 to 9 pounds, and are about 20 inches long at birth.

Lanugo and _____ , which protect the baby's body while stewing in amniotic fluid, begin to slough off in the weeks before birth.

    a. vernix
    b. cervix
    c. placenta
    d. Valtrex

A

a. Lanugo and **vernix**, which protect the baby's body while stewing in amniotic fluid, begin to slough off in the weeks before birth.

The lanugo (soft, fine hair that can cover almost all of the baby's body) and vernix (a white, waxy substance) that have been protecting your baby's skin have pretty much disappeared.

TIP Premature babies may still have quite a bit of this coating on them, while late babies may experience minor peeling of the skin. Both are normal and nothing to worry about.

9 MONTHS

It's a common misperception that babies are born _____ .

    a. with a silver spoon
    b. blank slates
    c. liars
    d. blind

A

d. It's a common misperception that babies are born blind.

Despite the widespread myth that babies are born blind, their vision is coming along just fine. In their last month in the womb, not only can they see, but they can also blink, swallow, and breathe.

9 MONTHS

Many fathers-to-be feel _____ ,
both confident and unsure of
their roles as dad and husband.

   a. excited
   b. conflicted
   c. nonchalant
   d. sad

b. Many fathers-to-be feel conflicted, both confident and unsure of their roles as dad and husband.

On one hand, you may feel completely prepared to be a father. On the other, you may be worried about whether you'll be able to handle your dual roles as a dad and husband.

9 MONTHS

You may find it hard to _____ after seeing what actual childbirth looks like.

    a. play the piano
    b. have sex
    c. sleep
    d. bathe

A

b. You may find it hard to **have sex** after seeing what actual childbirth looks like.

Childbirth is a wonderful thing, but that doesn't mean it always looks beautiful. If you've seen a graphic childbirth video in your prep classes, it may be hard for you to have sex with those images bouncing around in your head.

Even though society expects you to be strong and independent, you may find yourself feeling _____ .

   a. independent
   b. impervious
   c. unstoppable
   d. vulnerable

A

d. Even though society expects you to be strong and independent, you may find yourself feeling **vulnerable**.

Society expects men to be independent, strong, and impervious to emotional needs, especially during pregnancy. Most men, though, feel somewhat vulnerable and out of control, particularly toward the end of the pregnancy.

TIP Telling her about your worries and vulnerabilities will probably only worry or upset her. So find a friend who's been through it and spill to him.

9 MONTHS

First-time moms typically deliver as many as _____ their due date.

    a. 2 weeks before
    b. 3 days before
    c. 4 babies on
    d. 10 days after

A

d. First-time moms typically deliver as many as **10 days after** their due date.

Unfortunately, if your partner has been fixated on a specific due date, she may become frustrated and disappointed if that day passes and labor hasn't begun.

TIP If your partner is overdue, there's not much you can do besides pampering her as much as possible. Day spas can be great if they have experience with pregnant women. But she'll really appreciate a back or foot rub from you.

9 MONTHS

During the last few weeks of pregnancy, your partner is likely to feel _____ .

    a. happy and content
    b. hungry and sleepy
    c. miserable and uncomfortable
    d. angry and resentful

c. During the last few weeks of pregnancy, your partner is likely to feel **miserable and uncomfortable**.

If you put on 30 pounds, couldn't sleep, had constant back pain, had feet so swollen that you couldn't get your shoes on, and had something inside you stepping on your bladder every 5 minutes, you'd be miserable and uncomfortable, too.

TIP Encouraging her to rest, staying nearby as much as possible, and being calm and patient can help make things easier for her.

Women who stop working in the ninth month have a quarter the chance of _____ than those who don't.

    a. having a C-section
    b. winning the lottery
    c. writing a book
    d. needing an epidural

A

a. Women who stop working in the ninth month have a quarter the chance of **having a C-section** than those who don't.

Women who take leave in the last month of pregnancy have a C-section rate that is 4 times lower than women who don't take time off. That fact alone should be enough to get even the most workaholic moms to slow down.

TIP If your partner hasn't stopped working at this point, encourage her to do so.

If the baby is overdue, the doctor may order a _____ to be sure everything is still okay.

    a. nonstress test
    b. pregnancy test
    c. amniocentesis
    d. glucose test

A

a. If the baby is overdue, the doctor may order a **nonstress test** to be sure everything is still okay.

A nonstress test monitors changes in the baby's heart rate and movement in reaction to certain stimuli.

TIP This can get depressing for the mom-to-be and you. So remember the words of one OB: "In all my years of practice, I've never seen a baby stay in there."

If your baby is a boy, you and your partner should discuss whether or not to have him _____ .

    a. induced
    b. baptized
    c. circumcised
    d. circumvented

A

c. If your baby is a boy, you and your partner should discuss whether or not to have him **circumcised**.

There are many reasons, both for and against, that you should look at before making this sort of permanent decision for your son.

In the last month, many men begin _____ themselves for what their partner is going through.

   a. blaming
   b. applauding
   c. feeling proud of
   d. hating

a. In the last month, many men begin **blaming** themselves for what their partner is going through.

Yes, you got your partner pregnant. But she knew what she was signing up for when she agreed to have a baby. Don't torture yourself—use that energy to do something productive instead.

Younger women typically have _____ pregnancies than older women.

    a. harder
    b. easier
    c. longer
    d. shorter

d. Younger women typically have **shorter** pregnancies than older women.

In addition to age, several factors can influence due-date accuracy. For example, race can also play a part: African-American and Asian women tend to have shorter pregnancies than Caucasian women.

During _____ , contractions don't get stronger or more severe, and may eventually subside.

   a. real labor
   b. false labor
   c. cesarean section
   d. lactation

b. During **false labor**, contractions don't get stronger or more severe, and may eventually subside.

False labor contractions are irregular both in frequency and length. They may start or stop when your partner changes position (e.g., from sitting to walking, or lying to standing). Real contractions are often accompanied by aching in the back, abdomen, and pelvis, and they're relentless; changing position does nothing to slow them down.

9 MONTHS

Almost _____ of babies are born in hospitals, contrary to what you may see in movies.

    a. 50%
    b. 75%
    c. 85%
    d. 98%

A

d. Almost 98% of babies are born in hospitals, contrary to what you may see in movies.

While emergency births in taxicabs may be popular in movies and on television, in reality about 98% of babies are born in hospitals, and most of those nonhospital births are planned that way. Still, just about every couple worries about giving birth unexpectedly.

9 MONTHS

If your partner goes into labor and can't get to a hospital, the first thing to do is ____ .

    a. scream for help
    b. pop open a beer
    c. call 911
    d. tweet about it

c. If your partner goes into labor and can't get to a hospital, the first thing to do is **call 911**.

Operators should be able to talk you through what to do and will dispatch the paramedics right away.

Despite what you may have heard, you don't have to _____ to make him cry.

    a. take away a baby's toys
    b. slap the baby's bottom
    c. pinch the baby's cheeks
    d. insult your baby

A

b. Despite what you may have heard, you don't have to **slap the baby's bottom** to make him cry.

Babies don't need any outside intervention to get them to cry—they usually take care of that and the associated breathing by themselves. Of course, if he isn't breathing, CPR may be necessary.

LABOR & DELIVERY

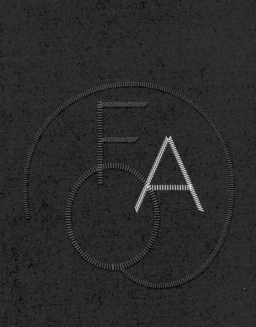

LABOR & DELIVERY

The entire labor process typically lasts _____ hours.

    a. 12–20
    b. 3–4
    c. 1–2
    d. 30–40

a. The entire labor process typically lasts **12–20** hours.

For a first-time mother, the entire process—from early labor through the birth of the baby—will take about 20 hours. For subsequent babies, chances are it'll be at least a few hours shorter.

_____ aren't allowed to perform surgery, and can handle only low-risk pregnancies.

a. Gynecologists
b. Pediatricians
c. Midwives
d. OB/GYNs

c. **Midwives** aren't allowed to perform surgery, and can handle only low-risk pregnancies.

Midwives are becoming increasingly popular in the United States as a more personal alternative to a traditional obstetrician. Keep in mind, however, that because they aren't MDs, midwives can't perform surgery, and they're able to handle only low-risk cases.

Women whose partners are present tend to have shorter
_____ .

a. patience
b. legs
c. labors
d. attention spans

c. Women whose partners are present tend to have shorter labors.

They also report experiencing less pain.

———

TIP Don't forget just how indispensible you are. Your active involvement during the birth of your child can make a big difference to your partner.

You'll need to be your partner's _____ when it comes to pain management during labor.

    a. doctor
    b. pharmacist
    c. advocate
    d. adversary

A

c. You will need to be your partner's **advocate** when it comes to pain management during labor.

As labor progresses, your partner will become less rational and less able to make big decisions. That means that you'll be the one making decisions about pain management.

TIP Discuss her wishes beforehand and keep them in mind. But be flexible. If an epidural isn't on your birth plan, don't argue with your partner if she screams for one.

In the United States, about _____ of women give birth using an epidural for pain relief.

    a. 25%
    b. 85%
    c. 60%
    d. 1%

A

c. In the United States, about 60% of women give birth using an epidural for pain relief.

Epidurals are by far the most common method of pain relief for childbirth. In some big-city hospitals, that rate exceeds 85%.

―――――

TIP Don't let anyone tell you or your partner what the best choice is for her; do your own research.

Epidurals are the most common type of _____ anesthesia.

   a. IV
   b. regional
   c. dental
   d. mental

b. Epidurals are the most common type of **regional** anesthesia.

Epidurals are typically administered during active labor. The medication will block the pain of contractions while leaving your partner awake and alert.

TIP "Awake and alert" is a relative term. By eliminating pain, an epidural will give your partner a well-needed break—and a great opportunity to take a short nap before the real work of pushing begins.

Some men may feel _____ if their partner chooses to use pain medication during labor.

    a. carefree
    b. angry
    c. disappointed
    d. jealous

c. Some men may feel **disappointed** if their partner chooses to use pain medication during labor.

You're supposed to be there to help her through the pain, right? So, the logic goes, if she needs to take pain medication, you're not doing your job or you've let her down (neither is true, of course).

TIP Lighten up and be thankful she didn't have to suffer. There are plenty of other ways to be helpful.

In recent years, giving birth
_____ (without pain medication)
has become very popular.

    a. loudly
    b. naturally
    c. quickly
    d. quietly

A

B. In recent years, giving birth **naturally** (without pain medication) has become very popular.

Just because natural childbirth (without drugs or medical intervention) is popular doesn't mean it's for everyone. Whichever way you go, make sure the decision is yours and your partner's (but mostly hers).

TIP Research all of the options, and support your partner's preferences—but build in some flexibility if something unplanned comes up.

During early labor, even though you're excited, you need to remember to _____ .

a. call everyone
b. eat
c. sleep
d. update Facebook

A

b. During early labor, even though you're excited, you need to remember to **eat**.

During early labor, if—and *only* if—your partner's OB says it's okay, she can eat light meals to keep her strength.

TIP Bring plenty of snacks (for yourself). She'll have hormones (and pain) to keep her going later; you won't.

LABOR & DELIVERY

If labor is progressing too slowly, the doctor may suggest using _____ .

    a. caffeine
    b. music
    c. Xanax
    d. Pitocin

d. If labor is progressing too slowly, the doctor may suggest using **Pitocin**.

In some cases, labor may be progressing so slowly that your partner may become too exhausted to push later on. In those cases, your doctor may suggest Pitocin, a drug that stimulates contractions, to help move things along.

LABOR & DELIVERY

_____ is used during labor to monitor contractions and the baby's heartbeat.

- **a.** Sonogram
- **b.** Electronic fetal monitoring (EFM)
- **c.** Contraction control machine (CCM)
- **d.** Underwater radar

b. **Electronic fetal monitoring (EFM)** is used during labor to monitor contractions and the baby's heartbeat.

There are two types of EFM: external and internal, both of which are harmless to the baby. If you watch the monitor closely, you can see contractions starting before you partner even begin to feel them.

TIP Resist the urge to say, "Uh oh, here comes a big one. . . ." You may think you're helping, but your partner will undoubtedly disagree.

If your partner is unable to walk or _____ during contractions, she's probably in active labor.

    a. laugh
    b. jump
    c. eat
    d. talk

d. If your partner is unable to walk or **talk** during contractions, she's probably in active labor.

Other hints include an aching back, fatigue, water breaking (if it hasn't happened already), and brown or bloody mucousy discharge.

During _____ labor, your partner's contractions will be 2–3 minutes apart.

- **a.** active
- **b.** forced
- **c.** early
- **d.** hard

A

a. During **active** labor, your partner's contractions will be 2–3 minutes apart.

These contractions will last 45–60 seconds, which doesn't give your partner very much time to recover in between. Pain will really begin to intensify, and she may become less talkative and more focused.

Encourage your partner to _____ during contractions and rest in between.

    a. cry
    b. scream
    c. punch
    d. moan

A

d. Encourage your partner to **moan** during contractions and rest in between.

The patterned breathing they teach in many childbirth classes isn't very effective in coping with pain. Instead, go for low, growly, guttural sounds, the kind you'd make if you tried to lift a car.

LABOR & DELIVERY

Verbally encouraging your partner during labor is _____ .

   a. pointless
   b. irritating
   c. remarkably effective
   d. just added noise

A

c. Verbally encouraging your partner during labor is remarkably effective.

When your partner is in labor, she needs all the encouragement she can get. And it means a lot more coming from you than from a nurse she doesn't know.

———

TIP Tell her she's doing great, and that you know she can get through this. You may be surprised at how effective such a basic approach can be in keeping her motivated.

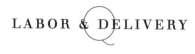
During transition, your partner's contractions may last as long as _____ .

   a. 10 seconds
   b. 90 seconds
   c. 5 minutes
   d. 2 hours

b. During transition, your partner's contractions may last as long as 90 seconds.

These contractions are pretty brutal and relentless, coming as little as 2 minutes apart. The pain is intense, and if your partner is going to ask for drugs, this is probably when she'll do it. She'll be tired, sweaty, and maybe even vomiting. Fortunately, this stage of labor is relatively short, lasting from 10 minutes to 2 hours.

LABOR & DELIVERY

The second stage of labor, push-ing and birth, is the most _____ .

    a. colorful
    b. calm
    c. enjoyable
    d. intense

d. The second stage of labor, pushing and birth, is the most intense.

Fortunately, it lasts "only" about two hours—although that's a word your partner would never use to describe what she's going through—and contractions gradually become further apart.

Another symptom of the second phase of labor is a loss of _____ .

   a. modesty
   b. blood
   c. temper
   d. feeling

A

a. Another symptom of the second phase of labor is a loss of modesty.

In phase one, the bed sheet may be up to her neck; in phase two, the sheet is halfway down; and in phase three, the sheet's all the way off.

LABOR & DELIVERY

As labor progresses, your partner may say something _____ to
you.

   a. hurtful
   b. funny
   c. loving
   d. sexual

A

a. As labor progresses, your partner may say something hurtful to you.

That may really tick you off—after all, you've been doing everything you possibly can to support her, right? But try to remember that the pain she's experiencing is extremely intense, and that she's trying to make it through the contractions.

TIP Just smile and do whatever she asks. She'll be back to her old self soon. Hopefully.

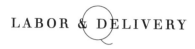
During labor, fathers experience a heavy dose of _____ pain.

   a. physical
   b. psychological
   c. imaginary
   d. empathetic

A

b. During labor, fathers experience a heavy dose of psychological pain.

While your partner is experiencing the physical pain of labor, you are most likely feeling plenty of psychological pain. This may produce an increased heart rate and/or a sudden adrenaline rush.

TIP It's sometimes easier for moms to recover from the physical pain of labor than it is for dads to recover from the psychological pain.

LABOR & DELIVERY

Once it's time for your partner to push, you may feel as though you're _____ .

  a. in the spotlight
  b. not needed
  c. ready for a beer
  d. ready for a nap

A

b. Once it's time for your partner to push, you may feel as though you're **not** needed.

At this point the medical team will step in and take over. That may leave you feeling helpless and, possibly, a little cheated. After all, you've been so involved up till now, that it doesn't seem fair to sideline you when the goal is so close.

TIP Let the medical team lead, but stay by her side and support her. They'll let you know what you can do to help.

Forceps or a vacuum may be used if the baby is in distress or your partner is too _____ to push.

    a. exhausted
    b. stubborn
    c. angry
    d. overweight

a. Forceps or a vacuum may be used if the baby is in distress or your partner is too **exhausted** to push.

The doctor may use forceps or a vacuum to help move the baby around and down the birth canal. This may sound scary, but it may help prevent the need for an emergency C-section.

The trip through the birth canal has probably left your baby with a _____ head.

    a. perfectly round
    b. square-shaped
    c. cone-shaped
    d. rectangle-shaped

c. The trip through the birth canal has probably left your baby with a **cone-shaped** head.

Don't worry, it's not permanent, and usually goes back to normal within a few days, if not hours.

In the United States, more than 30% of all children born in hospitals are delivered by _____ .

   a. FedEx
   b. nurses
   c. fathers
   d. C-section

d. In the United States, more than 30% of all children born in hospitals are delivered by C-section.

While expectant parents may expect and plan for vaginal delivery, sometimes things just don't go as planned. Worldwide, C-section rates vary widely, ranging from under 5% in Nigeria and other African countries, to over 40% in Brazil and several other Latin American countries.

Having an unplanned C-section can leave your partner feeling like a _____ .

   a. winner
   b. doctor
   c. failure
   d. mother

c. Having an unplanned C-section can leave your partner feeling like a failure.

She may feel relieved that the baby is safe, but may also be second-guessing herself and the decisions that were made.

TIP Be positive and reassure her that she didn't fail and that the decisions made—with the advice of medical professionals you both trust—were the best for the baby and her.

The placenta separates from the wall of the uterus during the _____ stage of labor.

    a. first
    b. premature
    c. third
    d. second

c. The placenta separates from the wall of the uterus during the **third** stage of labor.

Your partner will continue to have contractions as her uterus tries to eject the placenta and stop the bleeding.

LABOR & DELIVERY

One minute after birth, your
baby will be given a quick _____
test.

    a. blood
    b. IQ
    c. APGAR
    d. SAT

A

c. One minute after birth, your baby will be given a quick **APGAR** test.

The APGAR test measures Appearance, Pulse, Grimace, Activity, and Respiration. Your baby will get a score from 0–10 (2 points for each factor) and the test is repeated at 5 minutes.

TIP Yes, it's a test, but it's not a competition. Most babies score 7–9. No one gets a 10 unless the parents are friends of the medical team.

LABOR & DELIVERY

Anytime from 5 minutes to half an hour after the baby is born, the _____ will arrive.

   a. next baby
   b. uterus
   c. placenta
   d. hospital bills

A

c. Anytime from 5 minutes to half an hour after the baby is born, the **placenta** will arrive.

With all the excitement about the baby, most people forget that the birthing process isn't quite over. In most cases, the placenta, which is surprisingly large, will slip out on its own with a soft "plop."

TIP If this is an emergency birth, save the placenta in a bag, as the doctor will want to take a look at it when you get to the hospital.

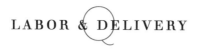
Some people believe that eating the placenta can help _____ .

   a. increase fertility
   b. make you smarter
   c. prevent postpartum depression
   d. the mother lose weight

c. Some people believe that eating the placenta can help **prevent postpartum depression**.

Consumption of the placenta is known as placentophagy. The placenta can be eaten raw, cooked, or dried. Research has so far proved inconclusive as to the benefits of placenta-eating.

TIP If you decide to do this, tell the nursing staff that you want to keep the placenta (no need to explain why). In many hospitals, placentas are routinely tossed out as medical waste.

LABOR & DELIVERY

Make sure to check your hospital bills, as _____ out of 10 of them contain errors.

    a. 9
    b. 7
    c. 5
    d. 2

A

a. Make sure to check your hospital bills, as 9 out of 10 of them contain errors.

Make sure that you and your partner check your birth-related bills carefully. Hospitals can make mistakes. In fact, a study by Equifax found that 9 out of 10 bills contain errors, rarely in your favor.

TIP Look for double billing or services you never received.

For months, and even years, after birth, your _____ may still be vivid in your mind.

    a. last date
    b. partner's pain
    c. doctor's face
    d. choice of hospital

b. For months, and even
years, after birth, your
partner's pain may still be
vivid in your mind.

When and if you decide to have
another baby, the thought of her
going through that again may
frighten you. She, however,
may have forgotten about the
whole thing.

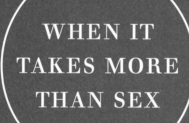

WHEN IT
TAKES MORE
THAN SEX

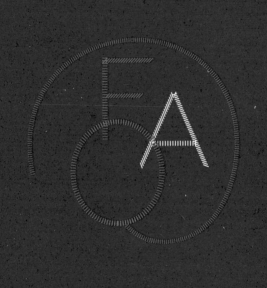

_____ can make you question your self-image and undermine your sense of masculinity.

    a. Your mother-in-law
    b. Lack of sleep
    c. Pregnancy
    d. Infertility

d. **Infertility** can make you question your self-image and undermine your sense of masculinity.

Infertility can do a real number on you, forcing you to confront shattered dreams, taking a terrible toll on your relationship, and even making you ask yourself how you could possibly be a "real" man if you can't get your partner pregnant.

As miserable as infertility may make you feel, it may be even harder on your partner, since society puts so much pressure on them to be able to have children.

_____ is not just a female problem—it can be traced to men 35–40% of the time.

a. Depression
b. Moodiness
c. Puberty
d. Infertility

d. **Infertility** is not just a female problem—it can be traced to men 35–40% of the time.

About 35–40% of the time, the problem can be traced to the woman. The same goes for men. For the remaining 20–30% of couples, it's a mix of his and hers issues or is simply "unexplained."

Smoking, drugs, medication, alcohol, and environmental toxins can all cause _____ .

    a. brain damage
    b. low sperm count
    c. weight gain
    d. mental illness

A

b. Smoking, drugs, medication, alcohol, and environmental toxins can all cause low sperm count.

Low sperm count or damaged/irregular sperm shape and movement can cause fertility issues.

TIP In many cases, low sperm count and other male fertility issues can be helped by simply making lifestyle changes, such as quitting smoking or adopting a healthier diet.

Only _____ of fertility patients need to use high-tech options like IVF and egg donation.

    a. 30–40%
    b. 3–5%
    c. 10–12%
    d. 20–25%

b. Only 3–5% of fertility patients need to use high-tech options like IVF and egg donation.

For those who don't conceive after all that, the remaining options are surrogacy or adoption.

Semen collection for analysis or artificial insemination almost always involves _____ .

   a. masturbation
   b. invasive surgery
   c. sedation
   d. injections

A

a. Semen collection for analysis or artificial insemination almost always involves **masturbation.**

There are a variety of ways to collect semen (either for analysis or artificial insemination), and if you close your eyes, you can imagine every one of them. In many cases, collection will happen at your partner's OB's office.

TIP If you'd rather not do it there, you may be able to produce a sample at home, as long as you get it to the lab within an hour. The advantage of doing it at home is that your partner can lend a hand....

Assisted reproductive technology (ART) refers to any _____ way of producing a pregnancy.

    a. nonsexual
    b. unplanned
    c. sexual
    d. consensual

a. Assisted reproductive technology (ART) refers to any **nonsexual** way of producing a pregnancy.

This includes in-vitro fertilization (IVF), donor eggs, donor sperm, preimplantion genetic diagnosis (PGD—usually done in conjunction with IVF), and surrogates (because the surrogate will likely be impregnated in a nonsexual way).

Ideally, during in-vitro fertilization (IVF), the lab will fertilize a _____ egg.

a. ripe
b. fresh
c. female
d. baby

b. Ideally, during in-vitro fertilization (IVF), the lab will fertilize a **fresh** egg.

A "fresh" egg is one that has just been retrieved from your partner (or a donor). Fresh embryos result in far more pregnancies and live births than frozen ones.

Men's fertility begins to decrease starting at around age _____ .

    a. 24
    b. 30
    c. 18
    d. 45

a. Men's fertility begins to decrease starting at around age 24.

The odds of conceiving within six months of trying go down 2% per year after that age.

When dealing with infertility,
sex can very quickly become
____ .

    a. hot and steamy
    b. routine and boring
    c. rare and expensive
    d. dirty and messy

A

b. When dealing with infertility, sex can very quickly become **routine and boring**.

At one point in your life, the idea of having sex every day may have seemed like a dream. But when dealing with infertility, daily sex can quickly move from hot and steamy to routine and boring. Having sex on a schedule can become a real chore, and sucks all the romance out of it.

About 25% of couples conceive in the first month of trying, and around _____ conceive within a year.

    a. 80%
    b. 60%
    c. 40%
    d. 50%

a. About 25% of couples conceive in the first month of trying, and around 80% conceive within a year.

In the middle, 50–60% conceive within six months and 60–75% within nine. If your partner doesn't get pregnant within a year, you're now in the black hole called infertility.

RESOURCES

Here are just a few resources to get you pointed in the right direction. You'll find a much more comprehensive list at mrdad. com/resources. If you know of a resource— or category of resources—that can benefit dads and their families, let us know: armin@mrdad.com

GENERAL

KIDSINTHEHOUSE.COM features 8,000 videos (including several dozen of mine) from more than 400 experts that can help answer all your questions on pregnancy and parenting. www.kidsinthehouse.com

PREGNANCYMAGAZINE.COM is one of the leading pregnancy websites. They publish 11 issues per year—including "The Pregnant Dad," the only pregnancy magazine issue written and edited by new and experienced fathers. www.pregnancymagazine.com

ADOPTION

NATIONAL ADOPTION CENTER offers a great list of questions to ask adoption agencies; addresses tax, single-parent, and legal issues; provides photos of kids waiting to be adopted, book reviews, lists of state and local contacts,

and links to other adoption-related organizations. Tel.: (800) TO-ADOPT
e-mail: nac@adopt.org   www.adopt.org

CHILDBIRTH

AMERICAN COLLEGE OF NURSE-MIDWIVES accredits midwife education programs, establishes standards, and provides information and referrals to midwives in your area. www.midwife.org

C-SECTION RECOVERY provides recovery tips, frequently asked questions, book and website reviews.   www.csectionrecovery.com

DOULAS OF NORTH AMERICA provides resources and referrals to doulas near you. www.dona.org

FATHERHOOD

CITY DADS GROUP is a growing, national organization dedicated to helping fathers socialize and support one another. www.citydadsgroup.com

JUST A DAD 247 has an amazingly comprehensive map of dads' groups all around the world—not just at-home dad groups, but all of them. www.justadad247.com/map-of-dad-groups

MRDAD.COM is my website. You can get information there about pretty much every aspect of pregnancy, childbirth, and fatherhood; find out more about my other fatherhood books; and send me questions and comments. www.mrdad.com

NATIONAL AT-HOME DAD NETWORK has great resources on how to find/register/start a dads' group. They also have links to stay-at-home dad bloggers, statistics, resources, and a lot more. www.athomedad.org

FINANCES

FAMILIES AND WORK INSTITUTE is a research and advocacy organization that produces a wealth of resources for working families and employers. www.familiesandwork.org

HEALTH

CORD BLOOD CENTER provides information for expectant parents and families considering cord blood banking. They are dedicated to finding the perfect option for your family whatever it may be. They provide the must relevant, up-to-date information on benefits, pricing, and current research for cord blood stem cells. www.cordbloodcenter.com

FIRST CANDLE offers resources on how to survive stillbirth and also guide you with decisions you need to make during this difficult time. www.firstcandle.org/grieving-families/stillbirth

MEN'S HEALTH NETWORK is a national education organization that recognizes men's health as a specific social concern. They have a fantastic database of articles, resources, and links on every conceivable fatherhood issue. www.menshealthnetwork.org

MORNING SICKNESS USA
www.morningsicknessusa.com

PREEMIE BABIES 101 is a parent blog inspired by the many diverse experiences that are common to parents of preemies. www.preemiebabies101.com

QUITDAY has some great information on the dangers to babies of cigarette smoke at home and in daycare settings. www.QuitDay.org

RESOLVE is a nationwide organization dedicated to advocacy and support for men and women with fertility problems.
Tel: (703) 556.7172   www.resolve.org

ABOUT THE AUTHOR

ARMIN A. BROTT, Mr. Dad, is a nationally recognized expert on parenting and the author of eight books on fatherhood, including the best-selling *The New Father: A Dad's Guide to the First Year* and *The Expectant Father: The Ultimate Guide for Dads-to-Be*. He has also written on parenting for the *New York Times Magazine*, the *Washington Post*, *Sports Illustrated*, and *Newsweek*, among many other publications, and he has been a speaker at the Dad 2.0 Summit. He writes the popular nationally syndicated column "Ask Mr. Dad" and hosts "Positive Parenting," a weekly syndicated talk show. Brott lives with his family in Oakland, California. To learn more, visit his website: www.mr.dad.com.

Please also connect with us on social media:

- @mrdad
- Facebook.com/mrdad
- Pinterest.com/mrdad
- Linkedin.com/in/mrdad
- plus.google.com/+Mrdad

OVER 1,000,000 FATHERHOOD BOOKS IN PRINT!

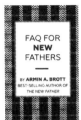
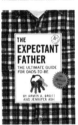
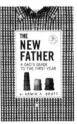